Breastfeeding Your Baby

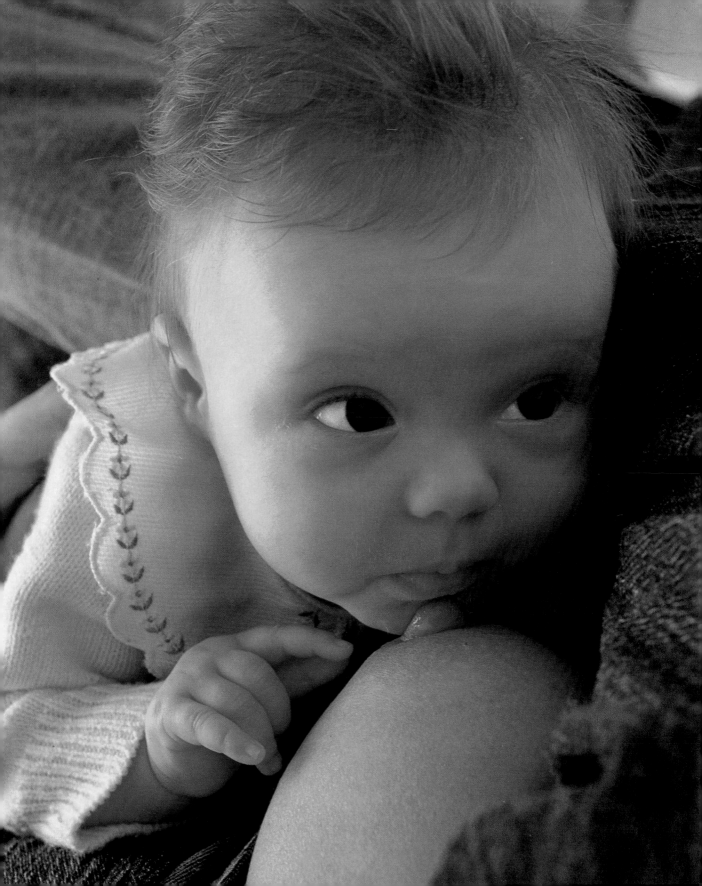

Breastfeeding Your Baby

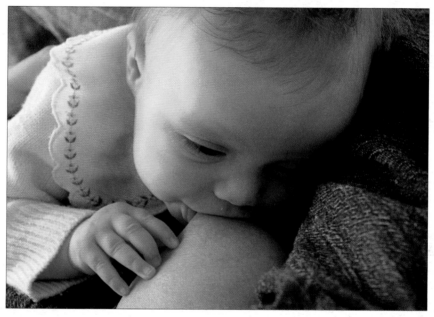

Sheila Kitzinger

Photography by Nancy Durrell McKenna
Breastfeeding Adviser Chloe Fisher

Alfred A. Knopf · New York · 1997

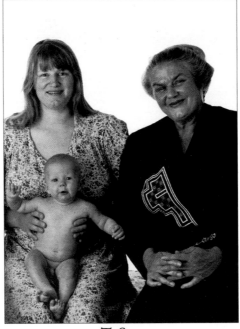

To Sam
and to my daughter Tess, his mother.
Thank you for teaching me so much.

A Dorling Kindersley Book

Art Editor Sally Smallwood
Project Editor Heather Dewhurst

Editorial Director Jackie Douglas
Art Director Roger Bristow
U.S. Editor Toinette Lippe
U.S. Consultant Gerrianne Griffin Bodd RN, BSN, CCE
This is a Borzoi Book published by Alfred A. Knopf, Inc.

Library of Congress Cataloging-in-Publication Data
Kitzinger, Sheila.
   Breastfeeding your baby.
   Bibliography: p.
   Includes index.
   1. Breast feeding—Popular works. I. Title.
RJ216.K58 1989 649'.33 88–27225
ISBN 0–679–72433–8

Published September 11, 1989
Reprinted Four Times
Sixth Printing, July 1997

CONTENTS

BREASTFEEDING YOUR BABY is a way of communicating intimately with another human being. It is never just a matter of technique, or of filling a baby with milk, as you might fill up the tank of the car with gas. It is true that there are techniques which are important, the most vital of which are those of helping the baby to get latched on well to the breast. But because breastfeeding is an expression of loving, it is also connected with your feelings. The techniques of breastfeeding cannot be isolated from how you are feeling about your baby and your body – whether you have confidence that it will work out, and whether or not you want to continue when there are difficulties.

Learning from the baby

It is sometimes said that those women who think about breastfeeding, and who read books about it, are the ones who do not succeed at it. It is certainly true that a woman's very determination may lead to her being so anxious that nothing seems to go right. But a great many of the skills of breastfeeding come not so much from instinct as from learning. This is mainly learning from the baby – understanding the baby's signals and responses, and being able to respond to them in turn. A baby is not just a little passive bundle, as any mother knows, but a living, sensitive being, who is learning and developing in her new environment and sending out messages from the very moment of birth.

Many women bring to the task of breastfeeding a very high idealism. By opening our eyes to how sensitive and aware a baby is, Dr Frederick Leboyer has taught us a great deal. But in some ways he has also had a negative influence, for when you see those smiling babies in his books and films – those little Buddhas with their inner radiance beaming out – you may feel that your baby should be like that too, and that if she is not, you are not a good enough mother. The truth is that there are very few babies who are in this state of beatific nirvana all the time. If you believe that your baby must never cry, and it is a sign of your failure as a woman and a mother if your child does cry, you will feel threatened every time she starts to assert herself as an independent being.

Having confidence in yourself

Breastfeeding is a psychosexual process, with all the hidden meanings that any sexual activity has for us. Like other psychosexual experiences, if it is to be satisfying it needs to be based on confidence and a sense of self-worth. Women often lack confidence. When anything goes wrong, we think that it must be our fault. When I was researching for my book *Woman's Experience of Sex*, I talked to women who had been subjected to violent sexual attack and who had been raped. They always asked themselves, "What did *I* do wrong?". Lack of confidence is endemic among women – certainly in Western societies, and perhaps the world over.

On the other hand, to many women the question that so many Western women ask, "Shall I be able to breastfeed?" or "Shall I try to breastfeed?" is rather like asking, "Can I breathe?" or "Can I walk?". Women in peasant societies do not talk about *trying* to breastfeed – they know they can. This became clear to me when I was doing anthropological field-work in the Caribbean. Jamaican women, who were often inadequately fed and who lived in poverty, all accepted that they could nurse their babies – and they all did. In industrial societies, however, breastfeeding has become a highly self-conscious activity. A woman feels the same anxiety as if she was facing an important examination.

Yet the free and generous flow of milk does not come from mental concentration. It comes instead from something that I can best describe in a French phrase, which translated means "being happy in your own skin."

In these pages I want to help you, through text and photographs, to acquire the technical skills of breastfeeding, and also to develop this relaxed self-confidence – so that both you and your baby can really enjoy breastfeeding.

A CHILD IS BORN

YOUR UTERUS has been for your baby a sanctuary and a nest for nine long months. You have felt feet kicking, head bouncing, body turning, knees twisting – all the energetic movements of a baby developing the neuromuscular coordination and strength to adapt to life in the world outside.

Inside the womb

Your baby has also been sucking inside the uterus. She has been drinking the amniotic fluid in which she floated and moved, and even sucking her fingers and thumbs.

She has been stimulated by practice contractions of your uterus (Braxton-Hicks contractions), by sounds she was able to hear from both inside and outside your body, and by the rocking movement of your pelvis as you walked and by the sudden rush of hormones in your bloodstream at times when you were highly aroused emotionally.

The onset of labor

Then labor starts. Contractions become firm squeezes and hugs which rise and fall in great waves of action. The hollow muscle in which she is contained embraces her so that she curls up into a ball, arms and legs flexed, chin tucked in on her chest. The contractions begin to press her down toward and then through the soft, dilated cervix, and slowly and steadily through the opening accordion-like folds of your vagina.

As she reaches the lowest point in the journey her face is downward, and the tissues of the posterior wall of the birth canal press against her face and in onto her nose and mouth. You push and she slides forward, edging little by little toward the light, and then sinks back as flexible tissues slip over her head again. You push once more.

The moment of crowning

At last the top of the baby's head reaches the opening and stays there once the contraction has finished. It is the moment of crowning. Her head is grasped by your muscles and you have a tingling, stinging sensation as if the head was encircled by a ring of fire. The pressure is powerful around the head while you wait for a message from deep inside your body to breathe – and push – and breathe again – and allow your baby's head to ooze forward to birth.

It comes slowly, steadily – all the tissues fanning open like the great petals of a rose as your baby surges forward and out. The head dips first down under the arch of bone formed by the front of your pelvis and then up, releasing the chin. Then the face slides up over your perineum. Water – the amniotic fluid to which the head has acted as a kind of stopper – now streams out and over the face. The head turns to come into line with the shoulders which are still inside you. Then they slide out and the whole body follows, slippery, wet, and warm.

Into your arms

You reach out to draw the baby to you. You hold and enfold this child whom you have only just seen, but who has been part of your body, part of yourself, for forty weeks or longer, and with whose movements you have become familiar as the beat of your own heart. This baby is new, but you have been companions on the same journey, and you trust each other. It is an emotional moment and you feel wonderful.

The baby turns his head toward your voice, selecting it out from every other background sound. The newborn is oriented toward the sound of the human voice, and – above all – to your own. The baby's eyes open and gaze at you steadily.

You feel the firm roundness of the limbs, the silky roundness of the head, and you stroke them in wonder. The newborn is sensitively responsive to touch. The baby relaxes. The long and difficult journey of labor has been to this home – the safe haven of your welcoming and protective arms.

The fetus may suck its thumb *and sip the amniotic fluid from the third month of pregnancy.*

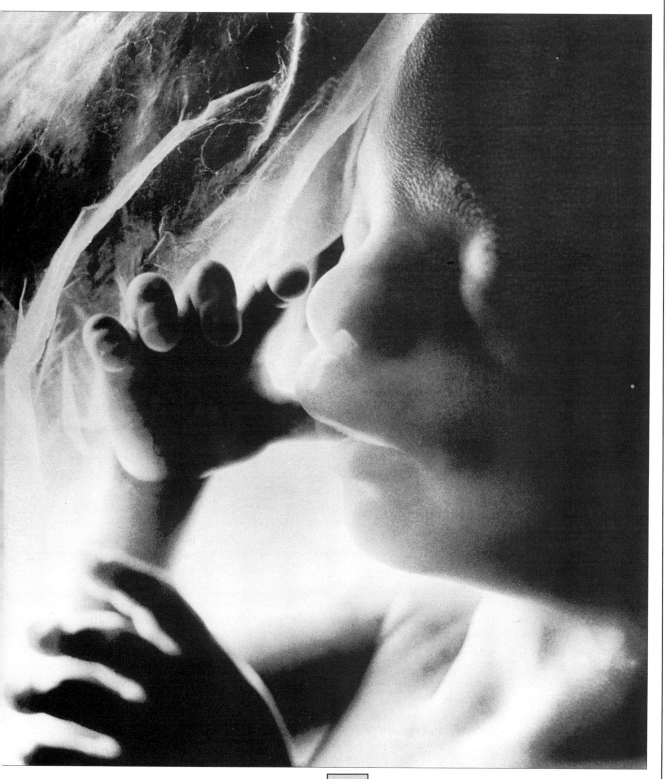

Benefits of Breastfeeding

IN DECIDING TO BREASTFEED you have made an important choice. The best way of helping your baby to grow normally and to give every possible protection against disease is to breastfeed *exclusively* for the first five or six months of life.

Nutritional value of breastmilk

Breastmilk is one of the most energy-dense foods in existence. Its ratio of protein, fat, and carbohydrate concentrations is uniquely adapted to the baby's needs and varies at different times in the day, even during a single feeding. When a baby is put to the breast, the first milk available – the foremilk – is low solute, so if she is just thirsty, a short suck will satisfy her. The longer a baby sucks from one side, the more fat and protein she obtains. It is impossible to arrange bottle-feeding so that the constituents of milk are adapted to the baby's needs in this way.

It is important to continue giving breastmilk after weaning foods have been introduced. A baby would have to eat a huge amount of cereal, sieved fruit, or vegetables before she was getting the level of nutrition available in breastmilk.

Benefits of lactose

Ninety per cent of the carbohydrate in breastmilk is in the form of lactose – milk sugar – compared with 4 per cent in cow's milk. In a breastfed baby the passage of milk through the intestines is faster than in a bottle-fed baby. Some of the lactose turns into lactic acid, which has the power to resist harmful bacteria, making bowel movements looser.

Lactose in breastmilk is less sweet than the sucrose added to cow's milk to make infant formula. So bottle-fed babies become used to a very sweet milk. Once any teeth come through, this can result in tooth decay.

Fat is more easily absorbed from breastmilk than from cow's milk. Babies who do not get enough essential fatty acids develop dermatitis, have a low blood platelet count which can result in hemorrhages under the skin, are susceptible to infection, and may fail to thrive. This particular combination of symptoms never occurs in breastfed babies.

Minerals and vitamins

Breastfed babies do not usually require any supplementary minerals or vitamins and giving them unnecessarily can be harmful. A healthy, well-fed woman makes milk rich in all the vitamins and minerals a baby needs.

Breastmilk is low in salt, potassium, and chloride. Cow's milk has three times as much. Babies do not need this heavy concentration of minerals, and excess quantities harm the kidneys. Breastmilk also contains a correct balance between calcium, phosphorus, and magnesium, important for growth and for bone development.

Breastfed babies are unlikely to be short of iron and zinc. These minerals are in cow's milk, too, but are less easily absorbed.

Resistance to infection

Breastmilk contains at least six anti-infective agents against the most common of childhood illnesses. A baby fed infant formula is four times more likely to get pneumonia, and nearly twice as likely to catch a cold. American bottle-fed babies suffer twelve and a half times more diarrhea than breastfed babies.

Antibodies against viruses as well as bacteria are present in breastmilk, protecting the respiratory and gastro-intestinal tract surfaces.

Two per cent of babies have an allergy to cow's milk. A baby with such an allergy who is started off with breastmilk may be able to tolerate some cow's milk after a few months. If there are allergies in your family, your baby will benefit from prolonged breastfeeding. She may still develop asthma and eczema, but the onset will be later and less severe.

One final benefit of breastmilk is that it is completely clean. Unless care is taken with sterilizing and making sure infant formula is made up fresh, it may be contaminated.

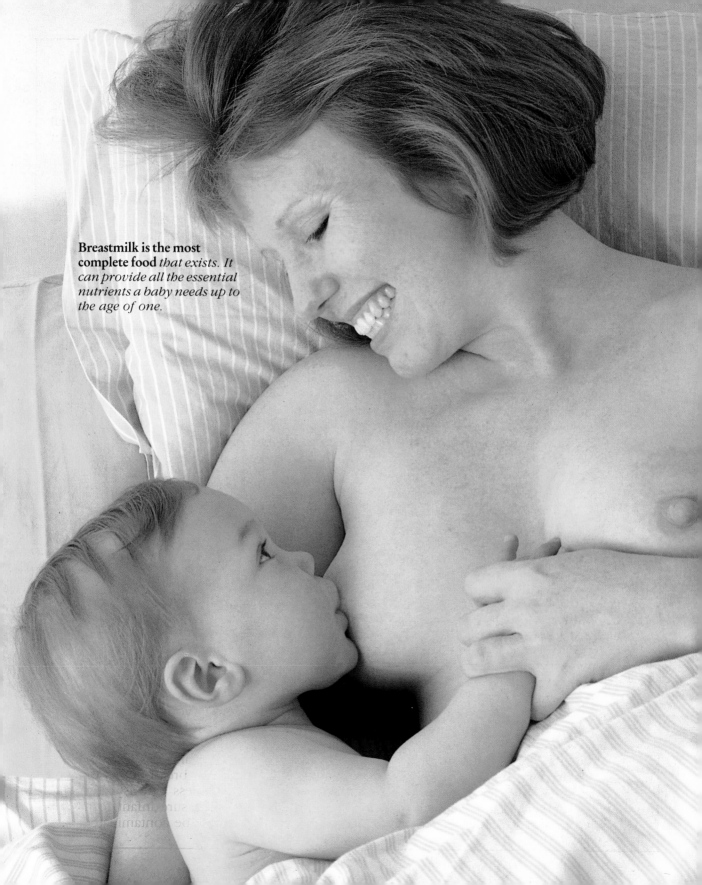

Breastmilk is the most complete food *that exists. It can provide all the essential nutrients a baby needs up to the age of one.*

Changes in Shape

Many women are anxious that breastfeeding will spoil the shape of their breasts. In fact, the really marked changes occur during pregnancy, not when breast-feeding. During pregnancy the area around the nipple – the areola – becomes darker, and the little bumps on it (known as Montgomery's tubercles) become more pronounced. As the glandular tissue increases, in order to make milk, the breasts become fuller and heavier and develop a looser, more generous curve. As a result, the nipples, instead of being centered, are now in the upper part of the breast globes.

These changes make it easier for the baby to nurse: she can nestle her chin into the lower part of the breast, get her jaw over the curve of the areola, and clasp the sinuses and glandular tissue firmly with her gums.

As breasts change their shape they can appear to sag or droop, and as this does not fit the soft porn image of breasts being firm and thrusting, we tend to see them as being less attractive than before. Yet this is the shape they need to be for a baby to nurse easily. Perhaps, instead of mourning our lost adolescent breasts, we can take pride in the way our bodies adapt so beautifully.

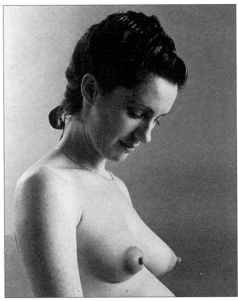

Your breasts become fuller *in pregnancy* (above). *When milk comes in, they swell so that the areolas are less prominent and become part of the breast's rounded shape* (right).

The shape of your breasts *adapts to the baby's needs in response to his sucking. After the birth, more blood is supplied to the breasts; on a fair-skinned woman the veins can be seen clearly, criss-crossing them like a network of tiny rivers and their tributaries.*

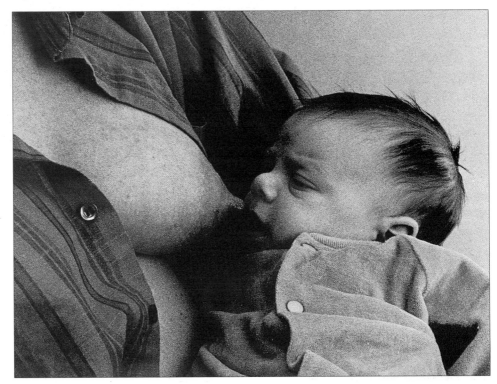

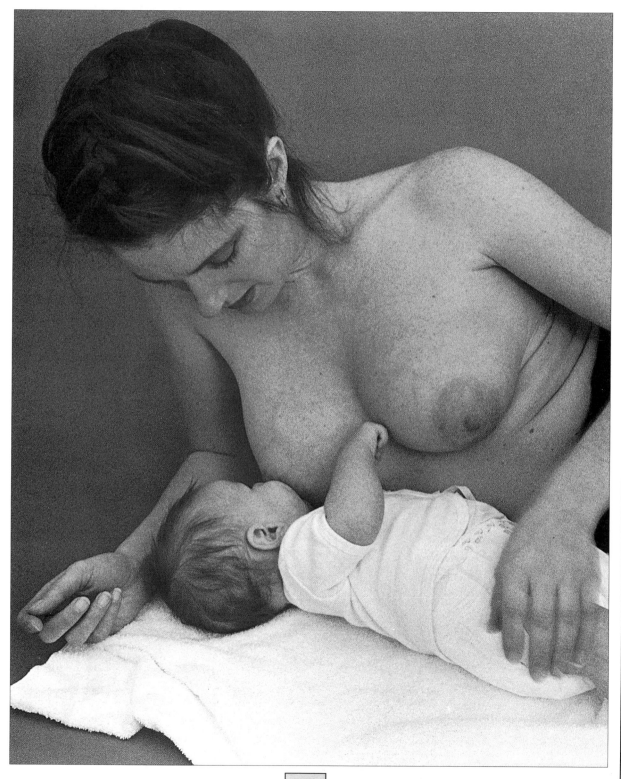

Types of Breast

Successful breastfeeding does not depend on the size or type of breast or nipple. There is no perfectly shaped breast for breastfeeding. Whether you have large or small breasts will not affect your ability to feed your baby.

Large breasts

If you have very large breasts it will be necessary for you and your baby to support them underneath while feeding. Otherwise the weight of the breast will drag it down and out of the baby's mouth, causing frustration for the baby and possible nipple damage. Also the lower part of the breast might not be drained well if it is not supported, which could lead to milk being impacted in the ducts and the breast becoming sore and inflamed (see pages 65–7 on mastitis).

A simple way of supporting your breast is to cup one hand underneath it. Alternatively, you can make yourself a sling out of fabric, and slip this under the breast and over your head, thus raising the breast slightly.

An ideal feeding position if you have heavy breasts is to tuck the baby under your arm so that her legs are pointing behind you, and cup her head in your hand.

Small breasts

If your breasts are small you may need to lift your baby up to the breast so that she can latch on. This is easily done by lying the baby on a cushion on your lap.

Breast surgery

If you have had breast surgery, some parts of the breast may not function as well as before and you will need to achieve good drainage of milk to prevent the breasts from becoming over-full. Even so, women who have had breast surgery often breastfeed with success.

Inverted nipples

Inverted nipples look a little like dimples – they point in instead of out. If you have inverted nipples, it will be harder for your

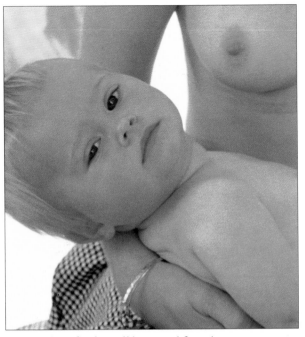

Most babies find small breasts *(above) easy to grasp, drawing the nipple to the back of the mouth and latching on to the breast's glandular tissue. If you have large nipples (below) it can be more difficult for the baby to get a firm latch, so make sure her mouth is wide open.*

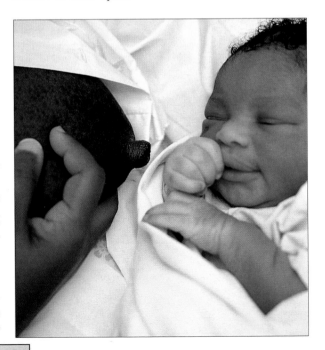

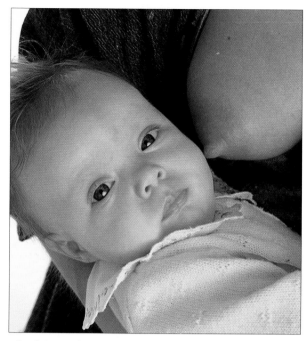

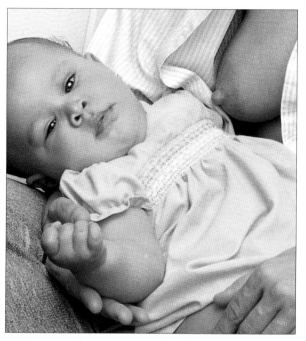

Nipples may be small *(above)* or large *(below)*. *Since the baby needs to suck at the breast, not the nipple, the exact size and shape is not important, provided that the mother knows how to help her baby latch on so that her jaw firmly grasps the breast's glandular tissue.*

Mothers may have small areolas *(above)* or large ones *(below)*, *but this does not affect breastfeeding. When a baby latches on and sucks at the breast, the action of the jaw molds the breast and nipples, which are composed of flexible tissue, to a shape and size to suit her mouth.*

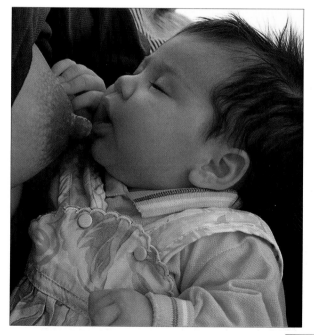

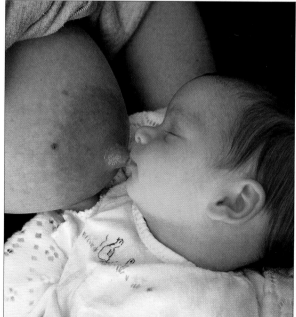

baby to draw them into the back of her mouth, and you will need patience and persistence in the first ten days or so to make sure that she gets a complete mouthful of breast every time she nurses. But her strong sucking will then shape and draw out the nipples so that they are adapted to her needs.

Women with inverted nipples often approach breastfeeding feeling they are bound to fail. Some women are even warned by people who are supposed to be helping them that their breasts are "no good" for breastfeeding, which of course places them under stress even before they lift their babies into their arms.

All nipples, however, change shape in response to the natural rush of hormones in the bloodstream. Falling in love with your baby and wanting to breastfeed involves just such a hormone surge. So your positive feelings about breastfeeding, your longing to hold your baby in your arms, your physical pleasure in the roundness of her head, her silky skin, her plump cheeks and tiny fingers, will all contribute to the physical changes that take place to enable you to breastfeed.

Remedies for inverted nipples

One simple way of producing a more pronounced nipple shape is to wrap several ice cubes in a face cloth, and hold this to your nipple, or keep a small plant spray filled with water in the refrigerator and squirt your nipples a few times before nursing your baby.

Another remedy is to circle the areola with a finger and lightly stroke the nipple. Or, if you need a stronger stimulus, use a breast pump to express some milk (see pages 138–9) before nursing. This will draw out the nipple and soften the area around it, making it easier for the baby to latch on.

The best remedy for inverted nipples, however, and one that gets at the cause rather than simply dealing with the symptoms, is correct positioning of the baby at the breast. Once you have got that right, the baby is in control and will mold your nipples to a perfect shape.

INVERTED NIPPLES

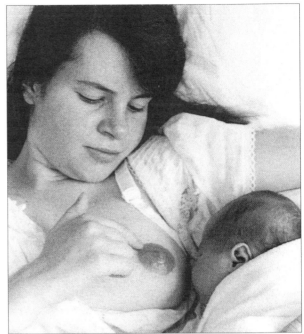

1 *Circle a finger lightly around the areola to stimulate the inverted nipple to emerge.*

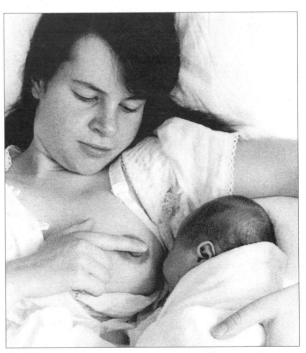

2 *Then stroke the nipple gently with your finger. It should become more prominent.*

If you have large breasts, *it is easiest to hold your baby between your legs so her head is level with your nipples. If your breasts are small, sit your baby upright.*

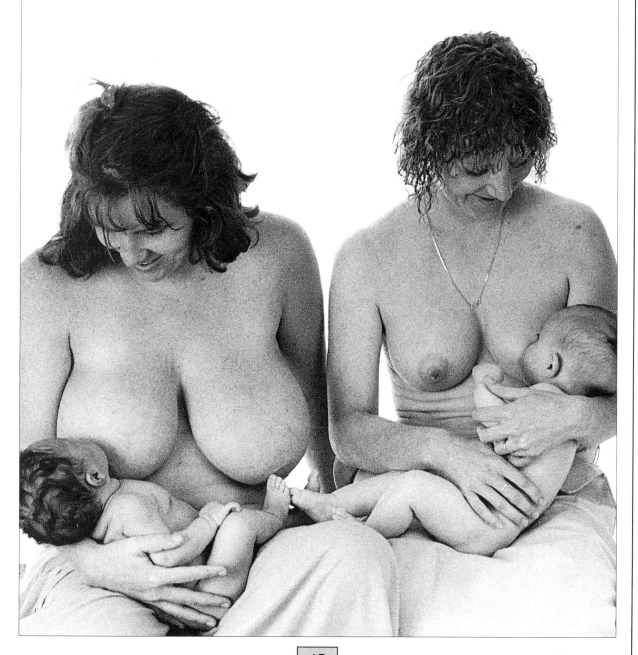

THE BABY COMES TO THE BREAST

The Minutes After Birth

THE IDEAL TIME to put your baby to the breast is within the first hour after birth. It is an important part of the way in which you welcome your baby into life and start to get to know each other. The baby's sucking reflex is especially strong during that first hour.

If this time is missed, a baby often loses all desire to suck for the next twenty-four hours, doesn't seem to have a clue when you try to put her to the breast, or may fuss and fret as if you were trying to force on her something particularly unpleasant. Giving a baby bottles during this time, even if they contain only water, also reduces the urge to suck at the breast. In some circumstances a baby may then have to be taught patiently how to latch on and suckle effectively.

Responding to your baby

On the other hand, you do not have to get your baby to the breast within a specified number of minutes of birth. There is no race to do it. Nor should it turn into a performance to show that you *can* do it, or a duty thrust on you by other people who want you to get it over quickly so that *they* can go off duty. The important thing is simply to watch the baby carefully and respond when she signals that she wants to suck.

As you hold your baby immediately after birth, you may notice that she starts to make sucking noises. As she looks around with evident interest at this new world, or gazes up in concentration at your face, she gets a bit fussed, as if there is something else she wants that would make it all perfect. She screws up her mouth, her lips twitch, she turns her head from side to side, and she may start to cry. These are all signals that she is ready to come to the breast.

Unfortunately, babies are sometimes already in their bassinets when all this is happening, so their readiness to suck goes unnoticed. But a baby in her mother's arms makes her wishes quite clear so that they can be acted on at just the right moment.

If your baby is very drowsy she may benefit from a little stimulation to help her find out what she wants. Cuddling, stroking and talking to her, and having her in skin-to-skin contact with you, provides this loving stimulation, and she will wake up and seek the breast when she is ready for it.

Triggering milk production

Putting a baby to the breast elicits a flow of two hormones – oxytocin and prolactin – which work together to stimulate milk production. Oxytocin causes muscle contraction and plays an important function in breastfeeding, as it squeezes muscles in the milk ducts and so leads to milk ejection. It also makes the uterus contract, so breastfeeding soon after birth helps the uterus tighten and prevents hemorrhage. Oxytocin is produced more readily when you are feeling good about yourself and experiencing physical pleasure. It has been called the "happiness hormone" and the "hormone of love". Holding your naked baby against your skin is part of the joy and sensuous delight in which this hormone works naturally for you, so that breastfeeding starts in a state of physical pleasure. The milk supply has to do with what is going on in our *minds* – with intense feeling and the power of emotions that flood our whole being – not only with technique.

Prolactin, the second hormone, has the specific function of preparing your breasts for milk production, and is secreted as a reflex response to the baby's sucking so that milk can flow. High prolactin levels usually prevent a woman getting pregnant when she is breastfeeding fully and frequently. Prolactin, in fact, is the most widely used contraceptive in the world – though it is not a reliable one.

Knowing that your baby can suck, feeling the strong tug of the jaw, realizing that you already have in your breasts the right food to sustain the life of your baby, makes a woman confident and strong in her mothering. It is a good way to start out.

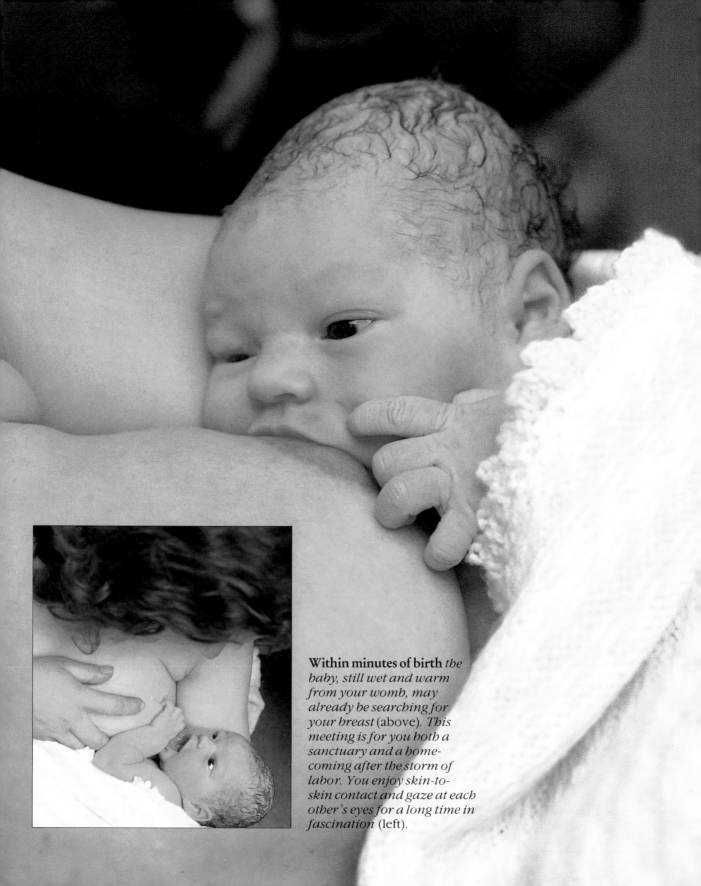

Within minutes of birth *the baby, still wet and warm from your womb, may already be searching for your breast* (above). *This meeting is for you both a sanctuary and a home-coming after the storm of labor. You enjoy skin-to-skin contact and gaze at each other's eyes for a long time in fascination* (left).

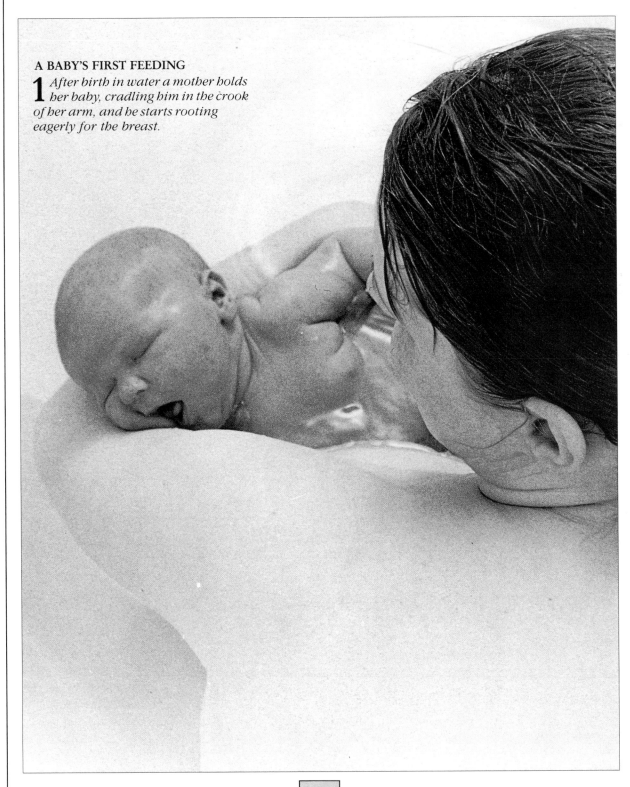

A BABY'S FIRST FEEDING

1 *After birth in water a mother holds her baby, cradling him in the crook of her arm, and he starts rooting eagerly for the breast.*

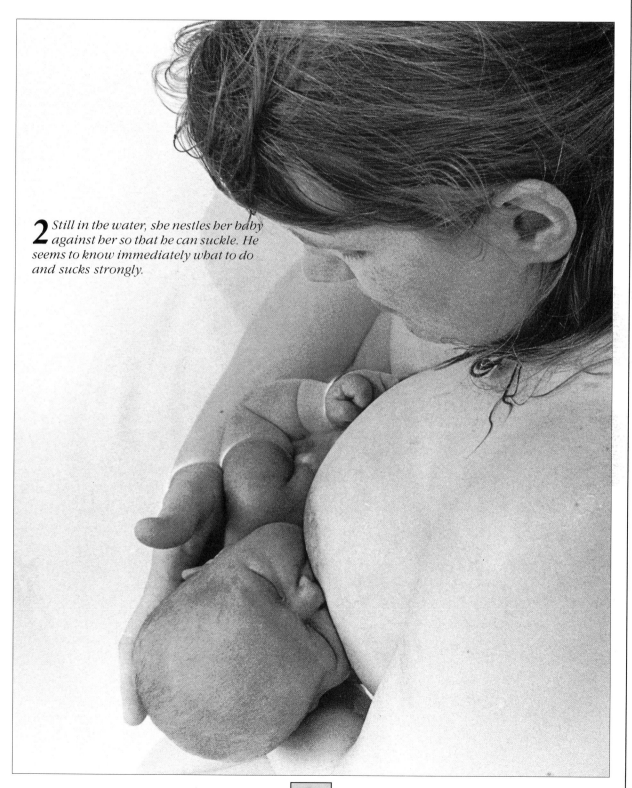

2 *Still in the water, she nestles her baby against her so that he can suckle. He seems to know immediately what to do and sucks strongly.*

The First Few Days

In the first few days after the birth you and your baby are both beginning to learn about each other – starting to get into step as if in the pattern of an intricate dance. At first there are bound to be some mis-steps in the dance, and when you notice them you change your behavior a little so that you find the rhythm again. As you start to develop confidence in your relationship with your baby, you will do the right things quite spontaneously.

Many of these rhythms you and your baby learn together have to do with breastfeeding. Though some babies take to the breast like ducklings to water, many have to learn exactly how to latch on if sucking is to be a satisfying experience. Mothers, too, usually have to learn how to help their babies best.

First milk

You may have noticed a slight dampness around your nipples in late pregnancy, or drops of moisture seeping from them if you were wearing a bra that was too tight and pressing on your breasts. This is colostrum, and is the first milk to appear in your breasts. Gradually, over the next few days, it gives way to mature milk. Some women express a little colostrum regularly in the last weeks of pregnancy, because they are told that this clears the ducts. There is no need to do it for this reason, but it may help you feel confident about breastfeeding if you can see that you actually have a working system. A few drops are enough.

Colostrum has unique properties. It is higher in protein and lower in fat and carbo-hydrate than mature milk, so the baby needs very little to get off to a good nutritional start. It also contains a higher proportion of sub-stances that protect the baby from infection. Even though your baby is getting only small quantities of colostrum, you are helping her to build up a strong immunological defense system. Colostrum is a laxative, too, ensuring that meconium in the baby's bowels is cleared out quickly. If this process is delayed, a baby

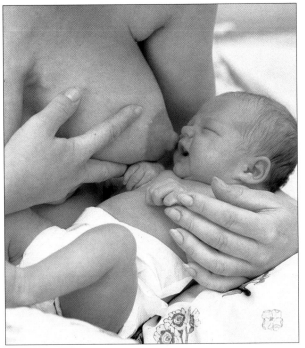

LEARNING TO BREASTFEED

1 *It may seem that your breasts are very large and the baby very small* (above). *You wonder how she can open her mouth wide enough to latch.*

2 *But she succeeds in latching on and sucks energetically* (right), *and together you begin the rhythm of breastfeeding.*

is more likely to suffer from jaundice, probably because meconium is reabsorbed through the gut walls.

Producing enough milk

It is important to resist giving any supple-ments to your baby in the first few days. Offering a bottle of infant formula or boiled water will reduce the frequency of sucking and the time the baby spends at the breast. Nurse whenever your baby asks for milk, and for as long as she wishes. Production and output of breastmilk is dependent on the frequency, intensity, and duration of sucking. So if you want to get your milk flowing well, and to produce a generous quantity, put the baby to the breast as often as you can.

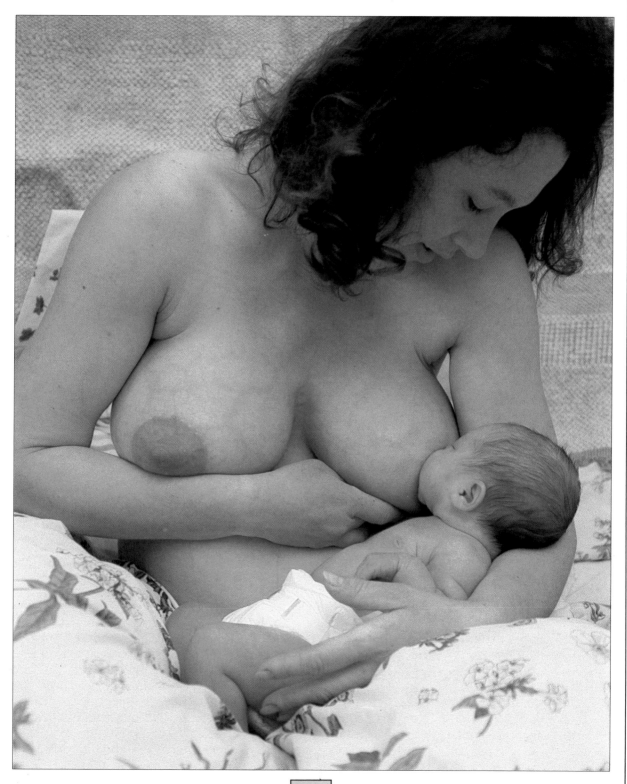

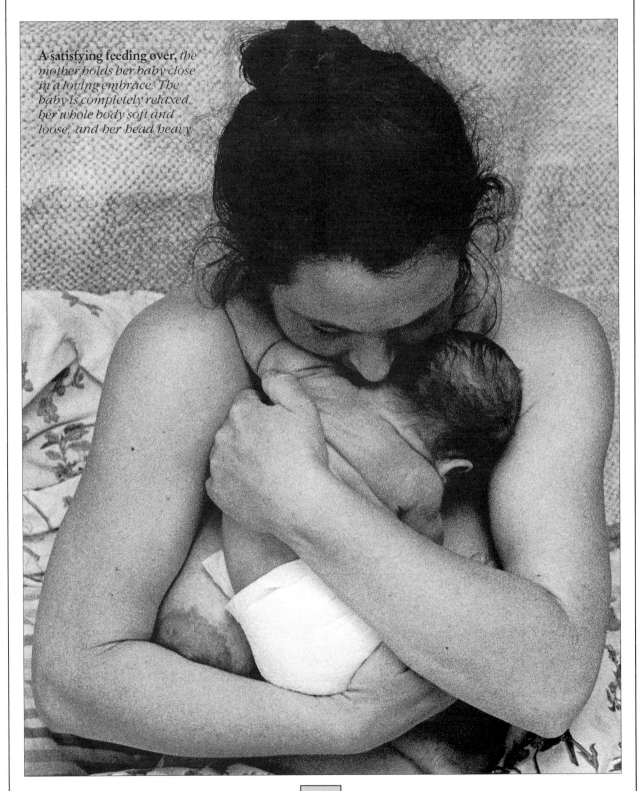

A satisfying feeding over, *the mother holds her baby close in a loving embrace. The baby is completely relaxed, her whole body soft and loose, and her head heavy.*

Stress can interfere with the milk ejection reflex and stop milk flowing well, so in the first few days especially, while you are still new to breastfeeding, relax and take your time:

• Select a peaceful setting.

• Find a comfortable position, with good back support.

• Do not hurry. You have all the time in the world.

• Pick up the baby *before* she gets fretful.

• Drop your shoulders, breathe out, and relax as you put the baby to the breast. While nursing, keep your shoulders and arms loose, and breathe slowly and regularly.

• Ensure that the baby is latched on to the *breast*, not just the nipple.

• Focus mentally on the visual image of your milk flowing into the baby.

• Have a glass of water or juice beside you to sip if you feel thirsty.

• If extraneous noises interfere with your focus on breastfeeding, create a musical barrier using your tape recorder or radio.

• Do not interrupt your time with the baby at the breast for anything or anyone.

• If necessary, take the phone off the hook, put a notice on your door saying "Mother and baby resting. Please do not disturb.", or have someone shield you from intrusions.

Your feelings

If your mother was unable to breastfeed you, or you do not have friends who have breast-fed easily, you may have many doubts about it and be concerned that you cannot produce enough milk. In many countries breastfeeding is still taken for granted, and women breast-feed not only because it is the safest and easiest way to feed babies, but because they have never seriously considered doing it any other way. In industrial countries, however, pregnant women often say that they will "try" to breastfeed their babies. They are pre-programmed for failure.

This is so not only because women often lack self-confidence, but because the manu-facturers of infant formula advertise "special" baby formulas with photographs of pretty babies thriving on their products. Nobody advertises a mother's milk. But that is, without doubt, the best milk for her baby, being exactly suited to her baby's needs.

Women often cannot trust their bodies to make milk. In many ways our bodies may have been a nuisance to us: when we have had to cope with the physical changes of adolescence, with menstruation and contra-ception, and, not least, pregnancy and birth. If the birth was complicated there are added reasons why we feel unsure about our bodies. But when milk starts to be produced and you can see it dripping out and the baby enjoying it, your body suddenly starts to make sense. This experience is especially important for any woman who has disliked her body in the past. Then breastfeeding comes to her almost as a revelation.

Fear of being drained

Breastfeeding may rouse very deep emotions. When the baby comes to the breast, latches on and sucks with vigor, it can feel as if you are in danger of being eaten up. Women who are having difficulties with breastfeeding often say they feel drained, and the baby is sucking out their energy. Yet the energy required to shop for, sterilize, prepare, warm and give bottles of infant formula, is more than that needed to lift a baby to the breast, cuddle her, and let your own milk flow.

The fear of being drained or consumed by the baby, however, often persists. Perhaps it has to do with the seemingly impossible demands for love and caring made on women – with being used up in nurturing other people, and having no time or energy for our-selves, and our needs.

When a baby kicks, punches, scratches, and bites you, you may feel you are being attacked, but it is important not to respond as if to an enemy. What you need to do is to show the baby that you survive these attacks, her fantasy destruction of you, and are still there – constant and unchanged. In this way you reveal to your baby what love is.

Nursing Positions

There are several different nursing positions you can adopt, and if you experiment you will soon discover which is the most comfortable for you. Whatever position you choose, it is important that you are relaxed as this will encourage the flow of milk.

The newborn baby

A newborn baby should be held to the breast so that she faces it full on. This will make it easier for her to latch on correctly. The best way to do this is to tuck the baby under your arm on the side you will be nursing, so that her legs are pointing behind you, and cradle her head in your hand. Then you can guide her gently to the breast. Alternatively, you can support the baby across your lap and hold the head with your free hand. Avoid putting pressure against the top of the baby's head, as this will make her lift her chin so that she is in a nibbling rather than a suckling position.

New mothers are often told to press the breast near the baby's nose to allow her to breathe. There is rarely any need for this, however, as babies' nostrils are conveniently flared, so that even when their mouths are stuffed full with delicious breast, they can continue to breathe. In fact, if you try to press the breast, it may accidentally push the nipple away from the back of the baby's mouth by deforming the sphere of the breast.

Once the baby is adept at positioning herself at the breast, it is not necessary to cradle her head in your hands and you can experiment with other positions.

Different positions

Most women nurse their babies while sitting in a chair, as this is the most convenient position. But you can also lie on your side with the baby next to you, which can be more comfortable if you have had stitches. Or you can sit cross-legged, thus forming a natural cradle for your baby. As long as you are relaxed and well supported, any nursing position is a good one.

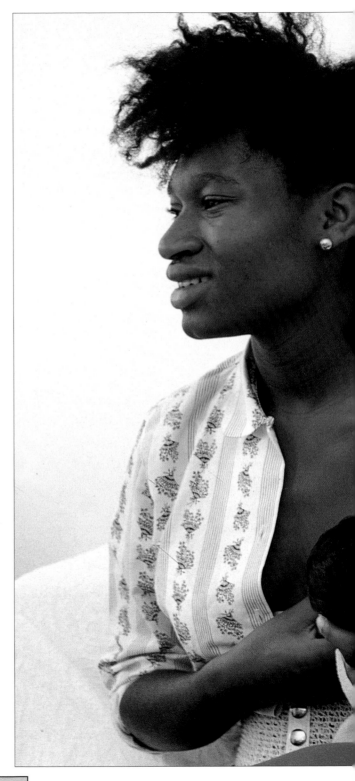

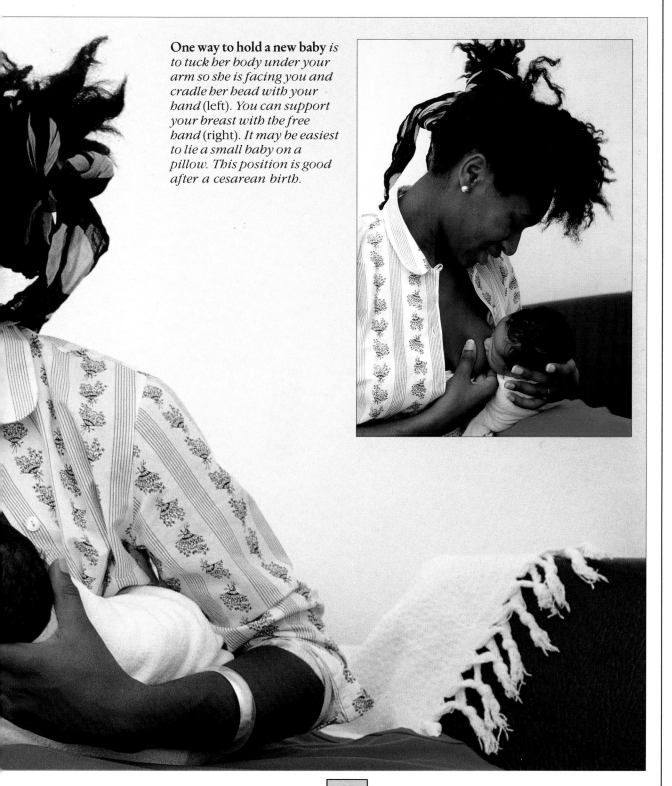

One way to hold a new baby *is to tuck her body under your arm so she is facing you and cradle her head with your hand* (left). *You can support your breast with the free hand* (right). *It may be easiest to lie a small baby on a pillow. This position is good after a cesarean birth.*

ALTERNATIVE POSITIONS

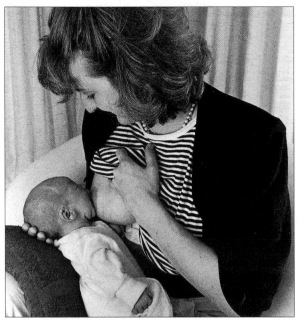

One way to nurse a tiny baby *is to place her on a cushion on your lap, and guide her head to the breast with your hand.*

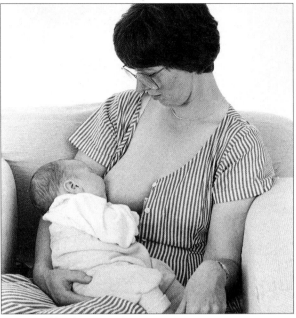

Sit a small baby upright *on your lap so that she can reach the breast more easily. Support her head and back with your arm.*

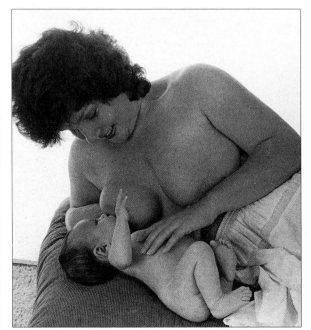

A semi-reclining position *is a good way to nurse your baby after a cesarean birth, but make sure you have pillows supporting your back and head.*

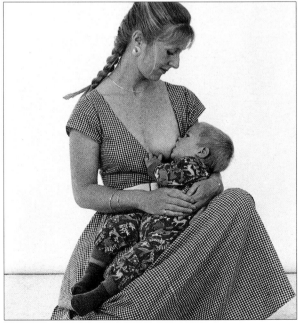

To nurse an older baby, *sit on a low chair with one knee raised higher than the other to form a natural slope for your baby to lie on.*

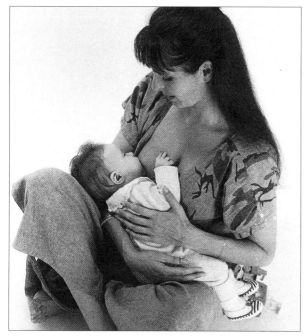

Sit cross-legged on the floor *and cradle your baby with both arms. This position is very comfortable and makes your baby feel secure.*

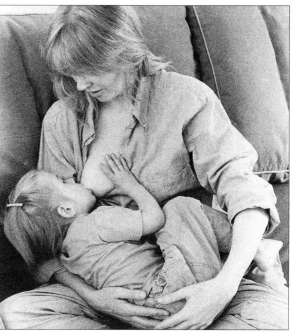

An older child will snuggle up to you *in a position comfortable to her. Sit against firm cushions for complete relaxation.*

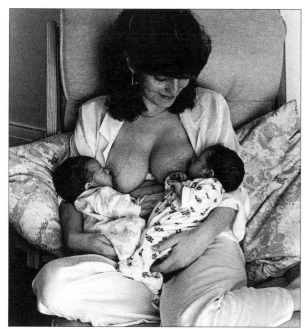

One way of feeding twins *is to sit comfortably in a chair with a baby at each breast. Make sure that your arms are well supported by cushions.*

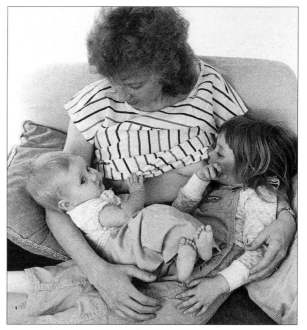

To nurse two children *at the same time, lie them across your lap so that the smallest child is on top of the other. Make sure you have firm back support.*

Latching On

The most important part of breastfeeding is knowing how to get the baby latched on to your breast. If you do that correctly, everything else follows naturally. Nearly all the problems women meet in breast-feeding – sore nipples, not having enough milk, engorgement, blocked milk ducts, mastitis and breast abscess, and a baby crying constantly with hunger – occur because their babies are not latched on well in the first place.

Finding the right time

Though most babies take to the breast quite naturally, there are some – equally intelligent – who don't seem to know what they are being offered and do not immediately latch on. And there are a few who even after they have latched on are slow to make the association between this and sucking.

As a general rule, babies will not respond positively to being put to the breast if they are very sleepy or if they are crying frantically. There is a special state of readiness for sucking, when the baby is alert and eager but not desperate. You will know it when you see it.

If some days have passed since birth and you still have not succeeded in getting your baby to enjoy the breast, you can start by feeding her expressed milk.

Feeding with expressed milk

Stimulate your supply of milk by sponging your breasts with warm water, gently massaging them, and expressing some milk every three hours or so (see pages 136–9). The exact timing is not important, but it should be done regularly.

THE LACTATING BREAST

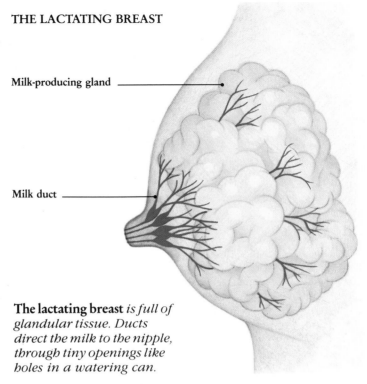

Milk-producing gland

Milk duct

The lactating breast *is full of glandular tissue. Ducts direct the milk to the nipple, through tiny openings like holes in a watering can.*

THE SUCKING EFFECT

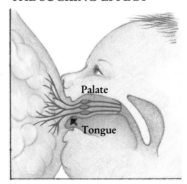

Palate

Tongue

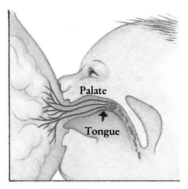

Palate

Tongue

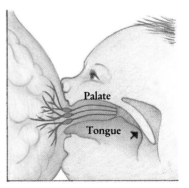

Palate

Tongue

The baby grasps the glandular tissue *with her jaw and presses the front of her tongue against the base of the nipple* (left). *Then the back of her tongue presses up against the palate* (below left), *which is automatically raised to seal off the nasal cavity, as milk flows down into her throat and she then swallows it* (below).

A GOOD LATCH

1 *A baby has powerful inbuilt survival skills and when ready for nursing seeks the breast with urgency and impatience, making movements that enable him to latch on correctly. With mouth agape like a hungry cuckoo, the baby comes to the breast, his breathing rapid and excited.*

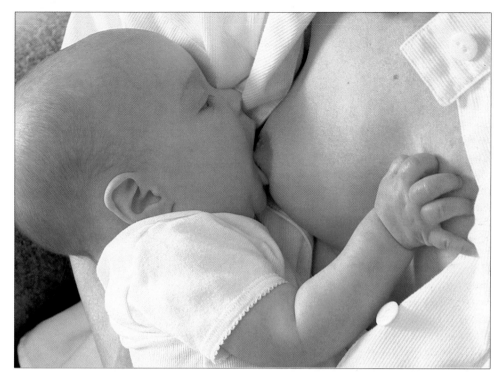

2 *Right on target, the baby clasps the breast with strong jaws so that the nipple slides deep into his mouth, and he feels the pleasure of the contact between the nipple and palate. Now that he is well latched on, he can suck vigorously to stimulate the flow of milk and the feast begins!*

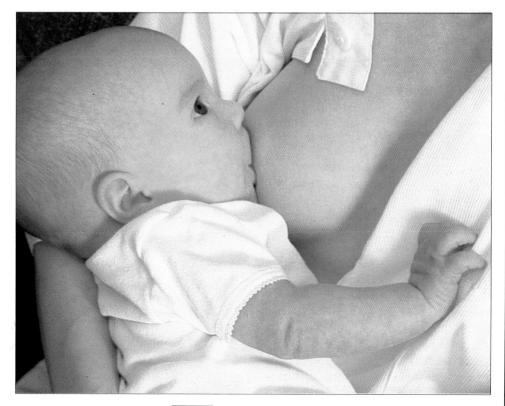

When you are ready to put your baby to the breast, first satisfy her initial hunger by giving her a little of your milk from a sterilized spoon or bottle. If you use a bottle, select a nipple shaped like a real nipple, so it will not surprise your baby to encounter the breast. Make sure that the hole in the nipple is not so big that milk pours out.

After she has taken about 1–2oz (50ml) of milk – not more – and is ready to stop for a moment, try putting her to the breast.

Helping your baby to latch on

Place the baby on your lap, her tummy against yours, and tease her with your fingers or your nipple, touching the sides of her mouth to let her know that something exciting is going to happen. Some babies will respond by rooting. Others will look as if they do not know what you are up to. Either way, watch for the moment when your baby opens her mouth wide, and then move her head firmly against the breast so that her bottom jaw holds the lower arc of the areola and the nipple slides in deeply, pointing to the roof of her mouth.

Patience and perseverance

If she latches, it is as if in one instant you have both got it right. If she does not latch, she will slide off easily. Then you do it again, and, if necessary, again, and again. ·

If your baby starts to fuss and cry, change her position radically, holding her upright over your shoulder or on her tummy on your lap, and soothe her into a state where you can start again. Talk to her reassuringly, letting her know by the tone of your voice that you are confident she will get it right.

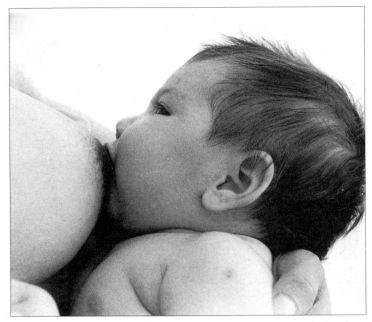

Wrong positioning *The baby is positioned too high on the breast* (above) *to latch on well. Her mouth is not open wide enough to grasp the breast tissues firmly so she is sucking at the nipple rather than the breast* (see below). *This will make the nipple sore, and the baby will soon be hungry again because she will be able to reach only the low-calorie foremilk, not the rich creamy hindmilk.*

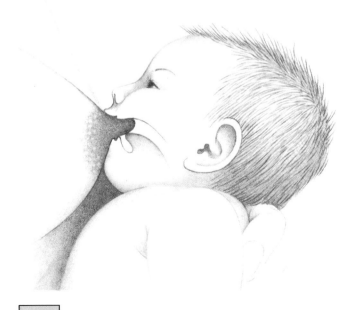

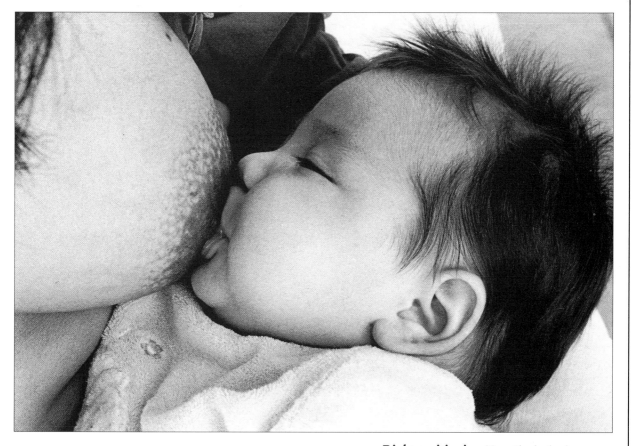

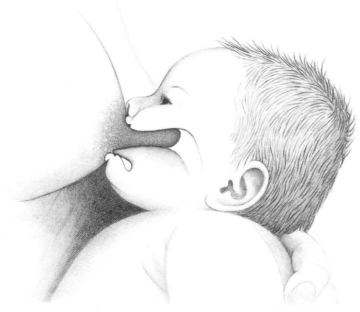

Right positioning *Now the baby has been repositioned and is latched on to the breast rather than the nipple (above). Her mouth is wide open and her lower jaw holds the lower arc of the areola. This enables her to get a good mouthful of breast so that she can pump the milk with her jaws and tongue from deep inside the breast. The nipple is drawn deep into the baby's mouth (left) so that it is pressed between the tongue and the palate, enabling her to suck well. This stimulates the milk ejection reflex and milk flows freely.*

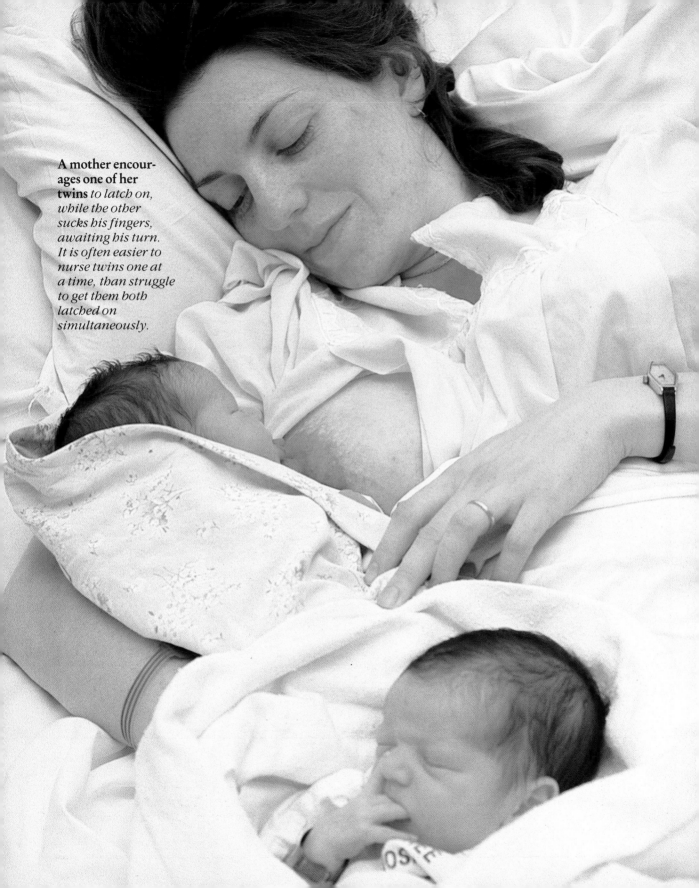

A mother encourages one of her twins *to latch on, while the other sucks his fingers, awaiting his turn. It is often easier to nurse twins one at a time, than struggle to get them both latched on simultaneously.*

BABIES AT THE BREAST

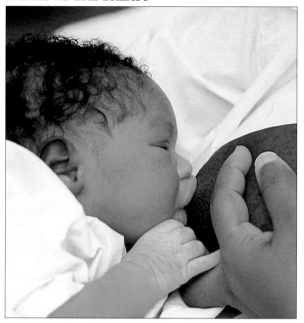

Oblivious to all *but the pleasure of warm, sweet milk, a baby who is well latched on to the breast settles down to a satisfying feeding.*

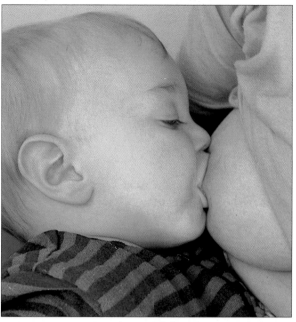

When experiencing the rush of milk *heralded by the milk ejection reflex, a baby is in a state of concentrated sensuous satisfaction.*

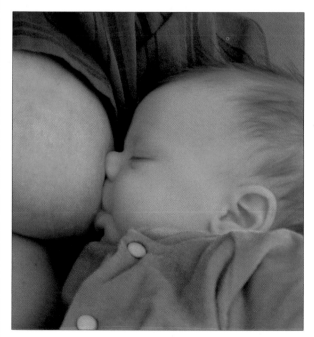

Babies are conveniently snub-nosed *and have flared nostrils so that they can continue to breathe freely when they are at the breast.*

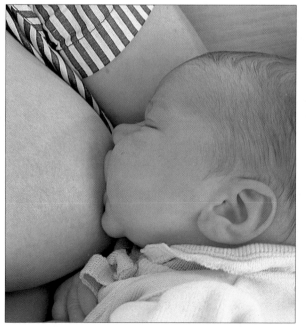

Babies also have receding chins *which makes it easy for them to fill their mouths with breast without any obstructions.*

Getting Help with Latching On

If your baby finds it difficult to latch on, you may want someone to help you put her to the breast. This could be your midwife, your partner, or a breastfeeding counselor.

First position yourself comfortably, either by lying on your side, supported by pillows, with your upper knee bent so that your back and shoulders are rounded, or sit up with your back well supported. For a right-handed woman, nursing at the left side is usually easier, at least to start with.

If your baby is not desperate to be fed, take a little time first for breast massage while someone else holds the baby and keeps her happy. Apply a comfortably hot towel to your breast for about fifteen seconds, then express some milk. Continue stimulating the breast until you can see drops of milk like pearls glistening on the nipple. Then you know that milk is ready and waiting for your baby.

The helper's role

Your helper sits at the same level by your side, facing you, and holds the baby so the heel of her right palm presses against the baby's upper back and shoulders, and her spread thumb and first finger of that hand supports the base of the back of the baby's head. With her other hand, your helper then lifts your left breast to the level of the baby's nose, and at the same time, with her right hand, guides the baby's head so it is facing the breast, with the mouth slightly below the level of the nipple.

In order to draw the lower arc of the areola and the nipple into her mouth, the baby has to lift her chin. It is impossible for a baby to open her mouth wide enough to latch on if her chin is *not* lifted, because then there will be insufficient space for vigorous jaw movement. As soon as the baby's mouth opens wide and the chin is well raised, your helper lifts your breast into the baby's mouth, introducing the nipple deeply, and tilting it *upward* so that it presses against the back of the baby's top palate. This entails careful timing and coordination of movement: the

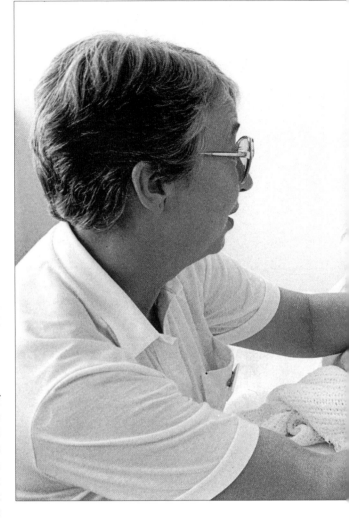

baby's open mouth has to meet the center of the breast at exactly the same moment as the breast is lifted into the baby's mouth.

While the baby sucks, the helper continues to hold the breast about 2 inches away from the areola, and presses in on the glandular tissue. If the baby has not latched on well, the helper moves her back in order to try again.

She may have to do this several times to get the latch right. Some babies are patient about this, while others get very cross. If your baby becomes furious, the helper should pick her up and cuddle and talk to her until she is soothed, before trying again. If she is crying and upset, *you* will get upset too, and she will

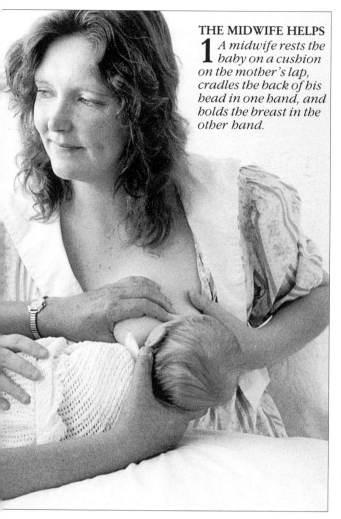

THE MIDWIFE HELPS

1 *A midwife rests the baby on a cushion on the mother's lap, cradles the back of his head in one hand, and holds the breast in the other hand.*

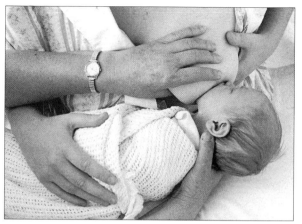

2 *She waits for his mouth to open wide, then latches him firmly on to the breast.*

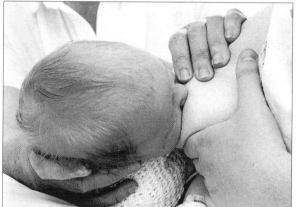

3 *The mother supports her breast underneath, well back from the areola, with one hand.*

be so angry that she will be too muddled to respond to the stimulus of the breast.

If the helper mistakenly presses on the areola, rather than the breast, the position is bound to be wrong. This results in only the nipple entering the baby's mouth. To suck well, a baby needs a good mouthful of breast.

Once the baby is in a good sucking rhythm it may be possible for the helper to remove her left hand from the breast and the baby will stay latched on. She will pause in her sucking occasionally and then continue as energetically as before. Let her go at her own pace. Talk encouragingly to her all the time and tell her how clever she is.

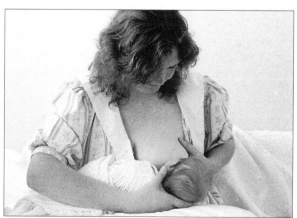

4 *Now the mother latches the baby on by herself, supporting his back with her right arm.*

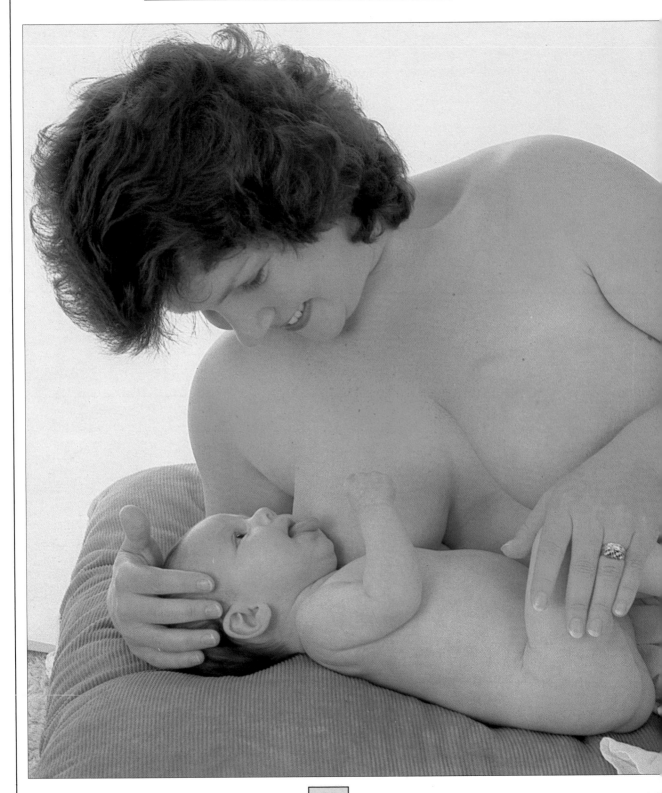

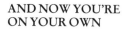

AND NOW YOU'RE ON YOUR OWN

1 *The baby enjoys lying naked* (left), *free to lick and explore her mother's breast. She gazes into her mother's eyes and her whole body becomes excited. The mother, in turn, gets pleasure from wooing her baby. Her breasts become hot and her nipples firm.*

2 *Now the baby actively roots for the breast* (top right), *turning her head from side to side and opening her mouth wide. The mother gently restrains an eager little hand so that it cannot get in the way, and allows her breast to drop into the baby's open mouth.*

3 *The baby latches on to the breast* (bottom right), *her jaws sealed tight, so that a vacuum is created. She draws the nipple deeply into her mouth and presses it against her palate. The muscles above her ears are working hard as she sucks with energy and vigor.*

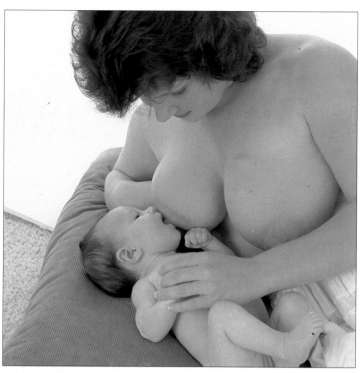

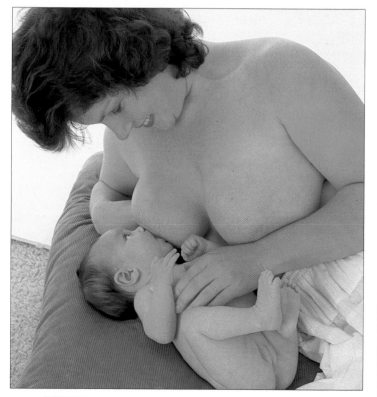

Sucking Rhythms

Imagine sitting down to a meal and having someone prodding you to keep chewing and swallowing non-stop. As soon as you paused to talk or to take a rest, this person would give your head a shove, smack your feet, bump you up and down or from side to side, or push the food impatiently into your mouth and tell you to get on with it and stop playing around. This is how nursing is for some unfortunate babies – no wonder they do not seem to enjoy it very much!

Sucking and swallowing

Each baby has an individual sucking pattern – it is not something you can force on a baby. But one thing is sure: no breastfed baby sucks and swallows without pause, except in short bursts, or at the beginning of a feeding when she is hungry or thirsty.

During a feeding there can be from three to fourteen "chomps," or sucks – two a second – and then a pause. The pauses last about half the time of the sucking, and are followed by another burst of sucking, and so on.

Fast flow of milk

When the milk supply is copious, for example at the beginning of a feeding, the baby swallows after each chomp, as she is trying to keep up with the fast flow. Or she may stop sucking entirely because milk is flooding her mouth and she needs to let it run out of the sides and down her chin. If she does not do this, she will gasp and choke on the milk.

The end of a feeding

When the milk ejection reflex is delayed, or the supply of milk is not so generous, and at the end of a feeding, there may be several chomps before the baby swallows. As a feeding draws to a close, a baby may have a snooze, wake up enough to have a few more chomps and swallows, and then drift off again, still with a mouthful of breast.

Babies often like to continue dozing and sucking intermittently for lengthy periods

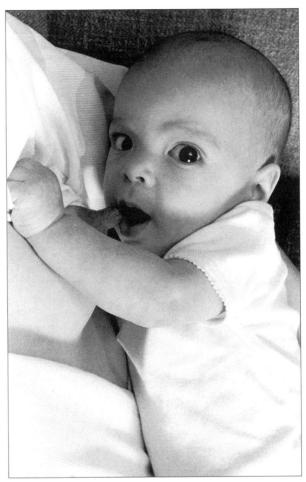

A baby pauses in mid-feeding *(above) to look around. He may smile at someone else, and notice interesting objects in the room. A baby at the breast learns that people are responsive – and that he can make them respond. Then he grasps the breast again and returns to nurse with fresh energy and enthusiasm.*

During another pause in feeding, *the baby looks up into his mother's eyes (right), his tongue still in the sucking position and his mouth full of milk. She smiles and speaks and he smiles and coos in return. Babies do not suck continuously without interruption. Once the initial hunger and thirst are satisfied there is time for a brief pause.*

after their hunger is satisfied. It feels so good to be at the breast that they do not want to let go. If you have other things you want to do, try putting her down with exciting objects to watch, or music to listen to. Or snuggle her up in a baby sling, or ask someone else to entertain her. You will soon learn what your baby likes best, and how looking in a mirror, having a bath, playing with a rattle, or being taken for a walk can mollify her for the temporary loss of the breast.

You may be aware that you have more than one milk ejection reflex during a feeding if, for example, it is interrupted for social reasons or because the baby needs her diaper changing, or she has a brief nap in the middle. You feel a second or even a third rush of milk,

and this will change the baby's sucking pattern as milk pours afresh into her mouth.

The pattern of sucking also varies between day and night. Fortunately, when you are rested and relaxed in the middle of the night, the baby is likely to suck regularly and be ready to settle down after a short feeding – especially if there is nothing exciting to attract attention. In the early morning, too, when you have a copious milk supply, she may suck in a businesslike fashion and then fall asleep again or else sit happily and play.

Social nursing

It is later in the day, especially in the early evening, when you may have the long leisurely feedings in which the baby clings to

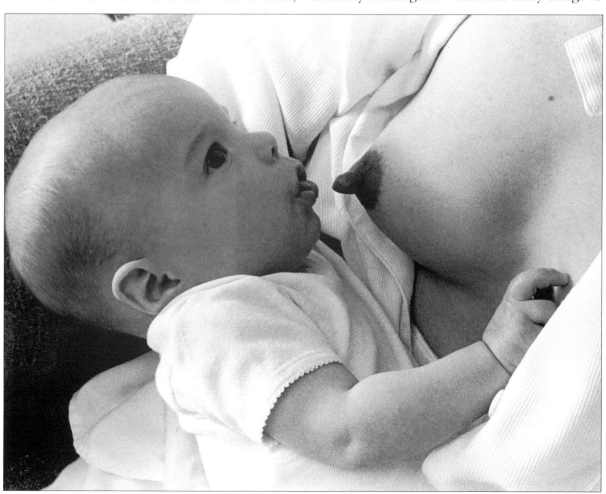

your breast like a barnacle on a rock. These feedings are characterized by quick-step bursts of sucking followed by an occasional swallow and then a doze. You may feel that you will never be able to prise the baby off the breast – even to go to the bathroom, answer the front door, or have some coffee. When a baby is adept at clinging on, come hell or high water, do not just pull her away or you will make your nipple sore. Instead, slip your little finger in the corner of her mouth to break the vacuum created by her sucking.

These lengthy feedings in which there are a variety of sucking rhythms are also the social feedings – ones in which a great deal of communication is going on between the baby and you. They are valuable for this reason. What is taking place is the start of language.

The baby slips off the breast, smiles at you, and then grabs the breast again. She pats your breast, or strokes the fabric of your shirt, then twiddles a button or zipper, or your other nipple, and looks up to see how you feel about these things. She comes off the breast briefly to inspect it visually, and then darts forward to grasp it in her mouth again. She fixes you with her gaze, sucking slows down, the nipple slips out of her mouth, and she coos and gurgles – but only for a moment. Then she homes in on it again and begins sucking vigorously. If you can be leisurely about one or more feedings in the day, you can both enjoy this social interchange.

Mother and baby dialogue

Breastfeeding is not all sucking and swallowing. It is about the exchange of thoughts and feelings – about being human. Mothers understand this well. While a baby is busy sucking, a mother is usually still and quiet, perhaps watching him and studying the concentration on his face. But when her baby pauses to look around or catch his breath, she starts to stroke, jiggle, or talk to him. Mothers and babies take part in a continuous dialogue, in which the mother is paced by her baby.

RHYTHMS OF NURSING

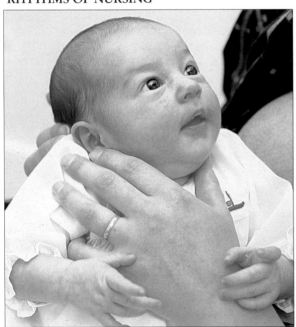

1 *When the baby slips off the first breast after a good, long suck, hold her upright to bring up any gas.*

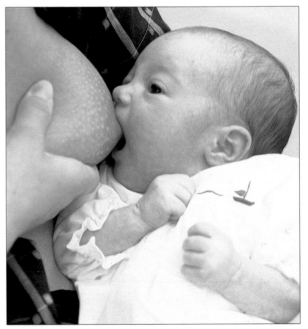

2 *Then offer her the second breast and let her suck as long as she likes at that side, too.*

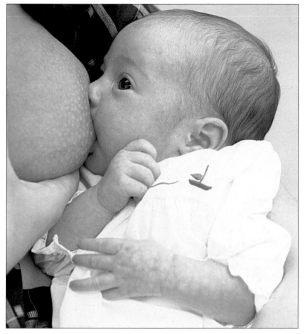

3 *At first she sucks strongly and rhyth-mically, but when she is getting full, the sucking slows down.*

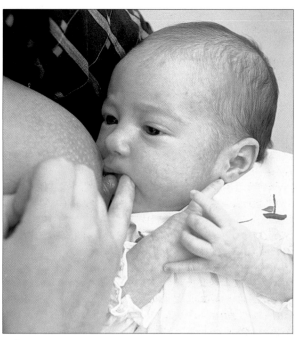

4 *If she is still firmly plugged on, but not sucking, slip a finger in her mouth to break the vacuum.*

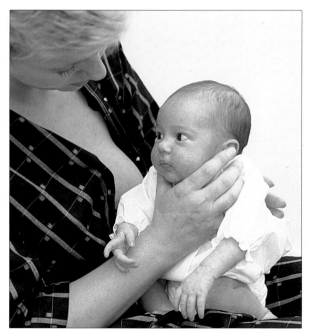

5 *Hold the baby in an upright position again and gently rub her back to see if she needs to burp.*

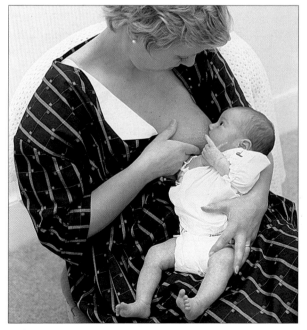

6 *After she has brought up some bubbles, it may be that she wants to have another suck at the breast.*

Nighttime Nursing

The easiest way to nurse your baby at night is to have him in bed with you. He will bask in the warmth of your body, and you can give the breast without delay whenever he is ready to nurse. This is less disturbing for everyone within earshot than waiting for him to cry.

It helps to have a wide bed, as you have more room for maneuver when nursing and will be more comfortable. Lie the baby directly on the mattress rather than using a pillow. There is no danger of suffocation for a healthy baby in a big bed – he will turn his head from side to side and move away if something blocks his nostrils and prevents him from breathing.

It has been suggested that babies benefit from the stimulus to breathing that comes from exhaled carbon dioxide – something they get only if they are close to other people, and that some crib deaths occur because babies sleeping alone don't have this chemical respiratory stimulus. Whether or not this is so, babies enjoy being cuddled up to a soft, enfolding body and they like to be able to reach the breast without fuss or delay.

If you choose not to have your baby in bed with you, you can keep him in the same room while he still needs nursing at night, so that you can reach him quickly. Obviously it is unwise for anyone to have a baby in bed with them if they are taking sleeping pills or other drugs, or have been drinking heavily.

Encouraging your baby to sleep

If you want to persuade your baby that nighttime is for sleep, rather than a lively social occasion, keep lights dim, avoid talking in a stimulating way, let your movements be slow and gentle, and stay drowsy and relaxed yourself – this may all come naturally, of course! – and unless your baby is soaking, or has a sore bottom, don't bother to change the diaper.

Some people cope well with disturbed nights and find it easy to fall asleep after nursing the baby, and wake refreshed after only a few hours' sleep. Others feel dreadful. If your partner is sleeping solidly while you have to wake two or three times in the night to nurse the baby, you may feel resentful and angry. After a week or so you may also be exhausted. Talk this over with your partner and suggest that he gives one of these feedings in the form of expressed milk from a bottle. This will give you an extra two to three hours' solid sleep and restore some much needed energy.

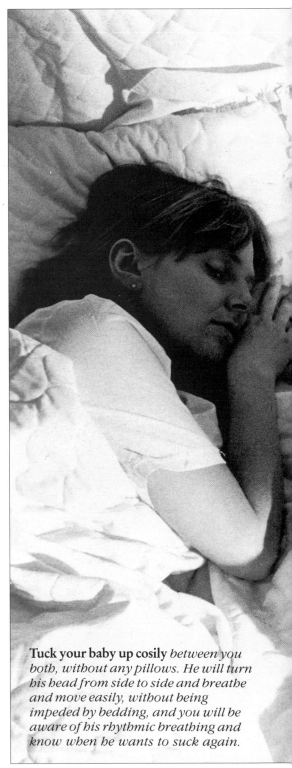

Tuck your baby up cosily *between you both, without any pillows. He will turn his head from side to side and breathe and move easily, without being impeded by bedding, and you will be aware of his rhythmic breathing and know when he wants to suck again.*

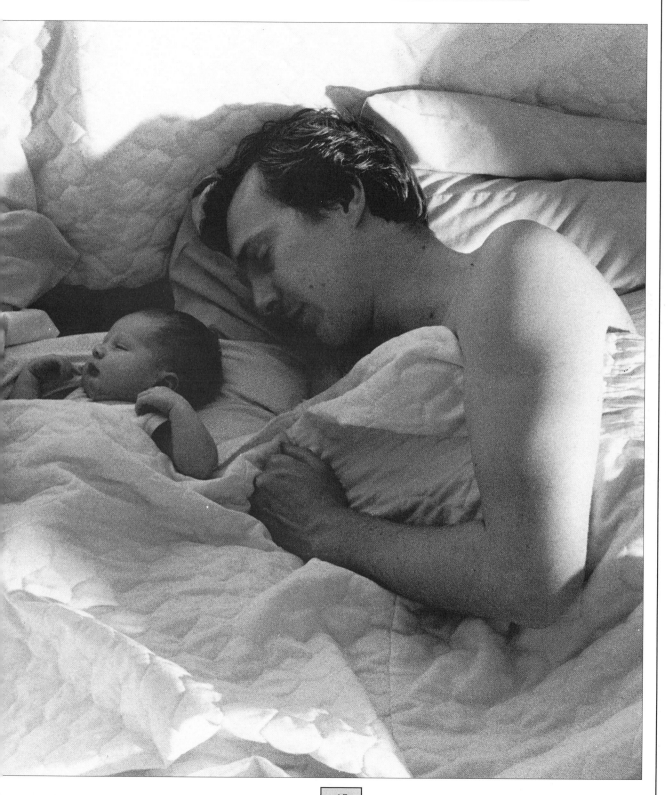

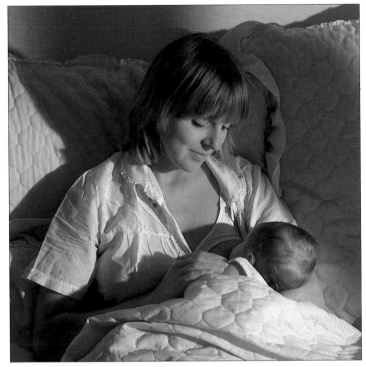

When you sit up in bed *to nurse your baby at night* (left), *make sure your back is well supported. It helps to have a pile of firm pillows against which you can rest. After you have finished nursing, throw the pillows out of the bed and tuck your baby up beside you.*

Your partner can take over *some of the night feedings* (below) *and offer the baby a bottle of expressed milk. This will satisfy the baby for an hour or two before he wants you, and it will give you a chance to catch up on your sleep.*

A relaxing way to nurse your baby at night *is to lie half on your side, supporting your baby in the crook of your arm* (right). *Since this is such a comfortable position, you may fall asleep with your baby still at the breast and wake to find him nestling against you.*

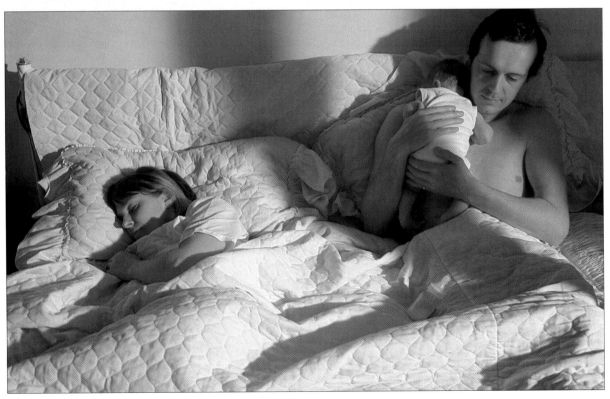

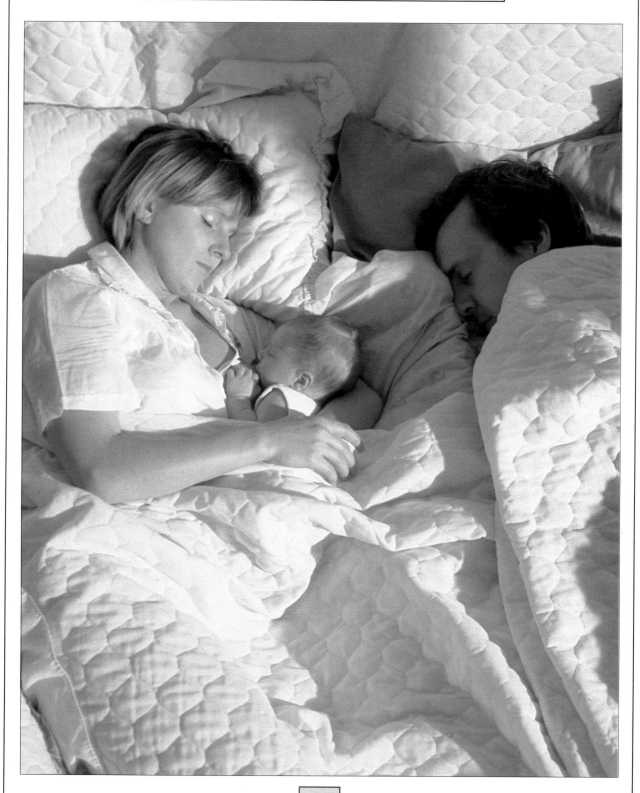

The Barrier of Clothing

It would not be practicable always to breastfeed naked, but if you do so occasionally, you will soon discover that clothing – both yours and the baby's – can act as a barrier to correct positioning of the baby at the breast, and turn the whole procedure into a juggling act.

From belts to bras

Wearing a thick sweater or a wide belt with a buckle at the waist can make it difficult for you to position the baby correctly against your body. A nightgown may not open up enough for easy nursing, and even those designed for maternity wear may bunch up in awkward places and get in the way.

Some bras can restrict and press in on the breasts so that even when you have managed to open the bra-flaps to nurse through, and struggled to poke your breasts through them, the globes of the breasts are distorted. A thick seam, or cups that are too small, may press on the breast causing continual leakage of milk and uncomfortably soggy nipples. Some bra fastenings, too, may be tricky to cope with one-handed. Tight-fitting clothing can press against the breast and make the nipple point at the wrong angle – instead of it being tip-tilted up against the baby's top palate, it goes in straight, as if aimed at her tonsils – making it difficult for the baby to latch on well. It can also prevent complete emptying of milk from the breast which could result in mastitis.

Going topless would appear to be the simplest solution, but as most people wear clothes most of the time, you need to have adaptable clothes in which you can nurse without fuss. Loose-fitting tops such as T-shirts and sweaters are the easiest things to wear. All you have to do is lift up your top and put your baby to the breast, without having to bother about undoing buttons or coping with awkward fastenings.

Baby clothes

Swathing your baby in layers of heavy clothing and a shawl will make it hard to position her correctly. An upturned collar, or rows of buttons or frills can all get in the way, while undershirts and sweaters can rumple up until they are bundled up round the baby's neck like a winter scarf, preventing her jaw from moving. The simple answer is to steer clear of fussy clothing and be careful not to overdress your baby.

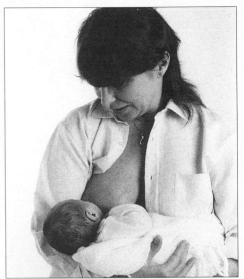

Wearing a loose shirt *makes it easy when breastfeeding. The fabric should be washable and preferably patterned so stains do not show.*

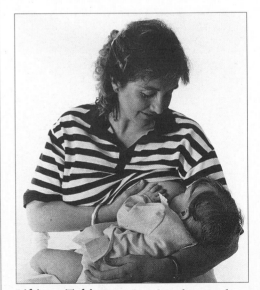

Lifting a T-shirt *involves less fuss and does not expose your breast, so it may be your choice if you want to breastfeed in a public place.*

It is lovely when you can breastfeed topless *and be in close skin contact with your baby. Even if you cannot do this all the time, you may enjoy the intimacy that comes when neither of you is impeded by clothing.*

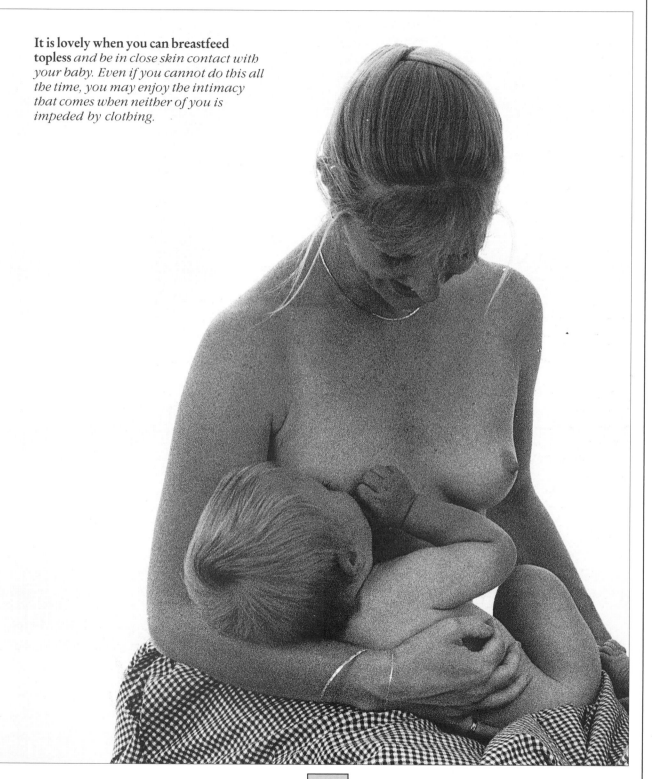

Feeding Yourself

WHEN YOU HAVE A NEW BABY you may find that you focus all your energy on the baby's needs and forget about yourself. As the weeks go by and you are busy coping with the phenomenal amount of laundry, cleaning, and constant tidying up that go hand in hand with a new baby, you may find that you skip meals or eat fast food because you are too tired to cook. When you are breastfeeding, it is very important to take care of yourself and to eat well, not only because the nutrients in what you eat pass through your milk into the baby, and not only because you have to be fit to look after a baby, but for your *own* sake, because *you* matter.

Eating sensibly

Special diets for breastfeeding mothers are rarely necessary. They omit valuable foods or put you under pressure to eat foods that you do not like. When you are breastfeeding you need to eat well – and should be able to enjoy your food. A combination of vegetable proteins, wholegrain cereal, fruit, vegetables and a small amount of animal protein makes the ideal diet. It is a good idea to eat some protein in the morning after you have gone eight to ten hours without food.

You will also need to eat regularly throughout the day as you may get very tired if you go for long periods without food. Snacks will help you maintain energy: a banana, some grapes or other fruit, a handful of nuts and raisins, a milk drink, a peanut butter, cheese or hummus sandwich, or a bowl of muesli may be the kind of thing that helps you keep up your energy level. If you are concerned about being overweight, keep a large bag of finger-sized raw vegetables in the refrigerator for you to dip into, and accompany them with some crunchy crispbread.

In the first three months when you are breastfeeding ad lib, it is best both in terms of your health and the baby's nutrition that weight loss should take place gradually. If you want to lose weight, delay going on a reducing diet until the baby is at least halfway through the first year of life. At that stage it is also a good idea to take up some vigorous physical exercise.

Avoiding certain foods

Some people may tell you that you should not eat certain foods because they will give the baby colic. All over the world breastfeeding mothers eat foods that in other countries are considered "bad" for the baby. If spices were the cause of colic, the entire infant population of India would be crying non-stop. If garlic contaminated breastmilk and made it unsuitable for babies, there would be incessant screaming in those countries situated around the Mediterranean.

Though it is worth watching to see if any foods you eat seem to affect the baby, most breastfed babies are able to tolerate everything in their mother's diet. If you are aware that you have a sensitivity to certain foods yourself, your baby may also be uncomfortable after you have eaten these things. Occasionally you might have to do some complicated detective work to discover if a food or food additive is upsetting your baby. Try omitting the suspect food from your diet for a trial week and then reintroducing it gradually and noting the result.

How much to drink

Breastfeeding mothers used to be advised to drink large quantities of milk, on the grounds that milk would make milk. This is rather odd reasoning as cows do not drink milk! They were also told to drink as much fluid as possible. You will probably discover that you want to drink more than usual, and it is a good idea to have a glass of water or juice beside you as you breastfeed. However, drinking large quantities of fluid in the evening may make your breasts very swollen and uncomfortable by the morning, and forcing yourself to drink excessive quantities of fluid ultimately *reduces* the milk supply.

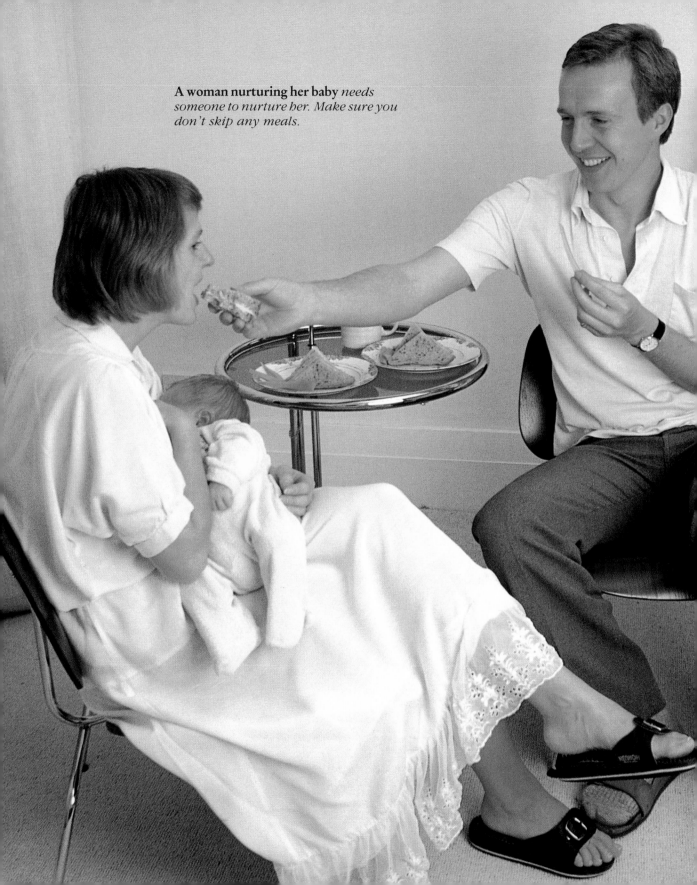

A woman nurturing her baby *needs someone to nurture her. Make sure you don't skip any meals.*

Fountains of Milk

In the first few weeks of breastfeeding, your milk may flow copiously and spurt out whenever your baby nurses, making her choke and splutter, and you feel you are awash in milk. After about four weeks, however, your milk production will settle down and be better adapted to your baby's needs.

Coping with gushing milk

If your milk gushes out, nurse from the less full breast first. When the milk ejection reflex begins, this will cause milk to spurt from the full breast, so that it is less overwhelming for the baby by the time she is put to that side. It can be difficult for the baby to cope with milk that streams out in great fountains if she is lying flat, so sit her almost upright to feed her.

Feeding may be a messy business to begin with so have a towel or tissues handy to mop up spills. Wear easily laundered clothing, and patterned rather than plain fabrics if milk stains are not to show. Cotton is ideal; silk and velvet stain badly. If milk oozes out between feedings, slip paper breast pads in your bra to absorb the drips, or press your elbows firmly against the outer margins of your breasts to reduce the flow.

Though it may be inconvenient, freely flowing milk is a natural safety device against blocked milk ducts, engorgement, stasis (congestion), infection, and breast abscess. Women whose milk drips and spurts rarely suffer any of these problems.

Collecting excess milk

If you are organized, you can collect your excess milk and build up a store in the freezer for when you are away from your baby. Alternatively, you may be able to give it to a milk bank at your local hospital. Check with your pediatrician to find out how do to this.

You will need a sterilized bottle, lid, and nipple shield. Suitable shields can be obtained from a lactation consultant. (For details on sterilizing, see page 138.) Place a shield over the breast from which you will not be nursing. When the baby begins to nurse, milk will drip and sometimes even pour into the shield. At the end of nursing, tip the milk from the shield into the sterilized bottle, put the lid on, and place it in the refrigerator. You can add more milk to the bottle throughout the day, but after twenty-four hours it should be put in the freezer.

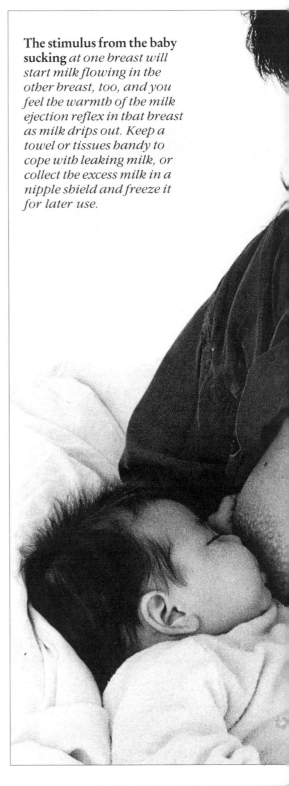

The stimulus from the baby sucking *at one breast will start milk flowing in the other breast, too, and you feel the warmth of the milk ejection reflex in that breast as milk drips out. Keep a towel or tissues handy to cope with leaking milk, or collect the excess milk in a nipple shield and freeze it for later use.*

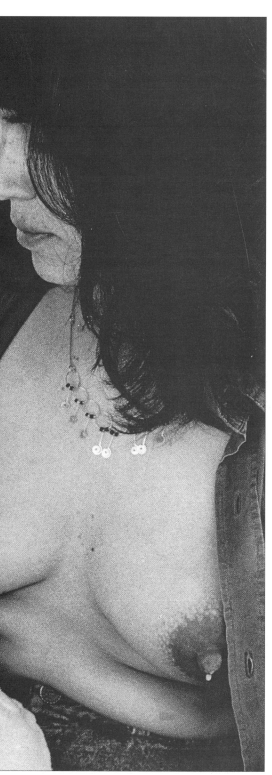

THE MILK EJECTION REFLEX

The baby's sucking stimulates nerve endings in the areola which pass the message to the pituitary gland in the brain.

Pituitary gland

The pituitary gland produces oxytocin and prolactin which cause the muscle wall of the milk-producing glands to contract so that the milk spurts out.

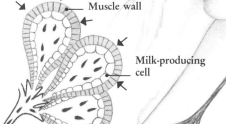

Milk-producing gland

Muscle wall

Milk-producing cell

Milk duct

Milk-producing glands

As your baby latches on, *nerve endings in your breast are stimulated to send a signal to the hypothalamus – a part of the brain that controls metabolism. This in turn signals to the pituitary gland to release oxytocin and prolactin, the hormones concerned with making and releasing milk. Shortly after*

your baby has begun to suck, these hormones cause the muscle walls of the milk-producing glands to contract, so that the cells lining the glands squeeze milk into the milk ducts. The milk rushes down the ducts to the nipple and into the baby's mouth. This is known as the milk ejection reflex.

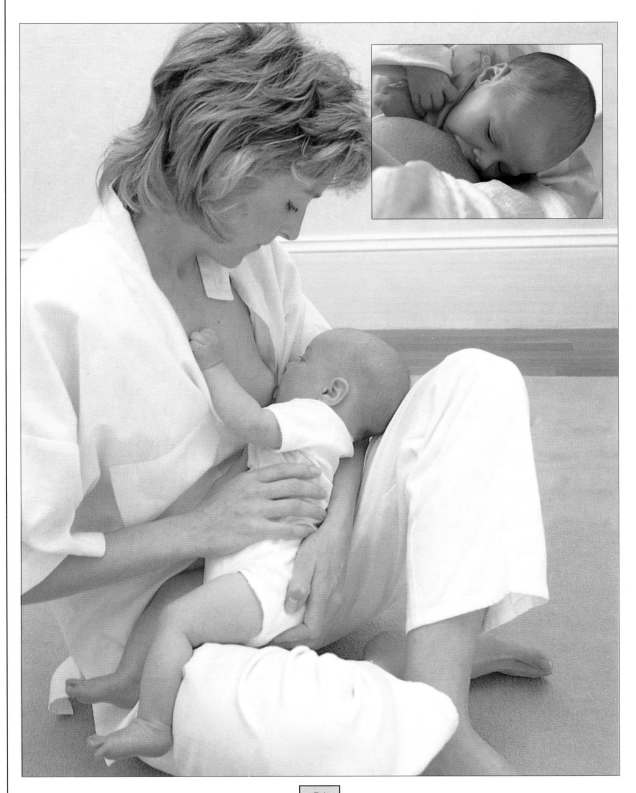

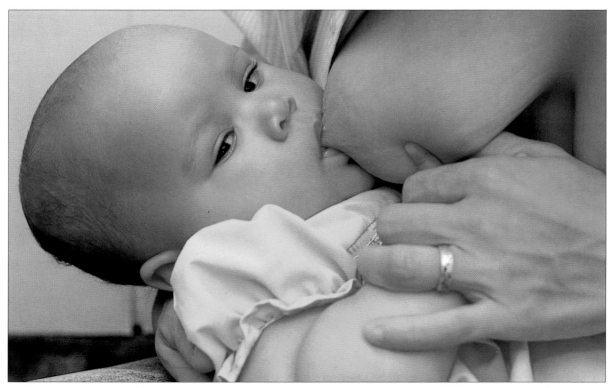

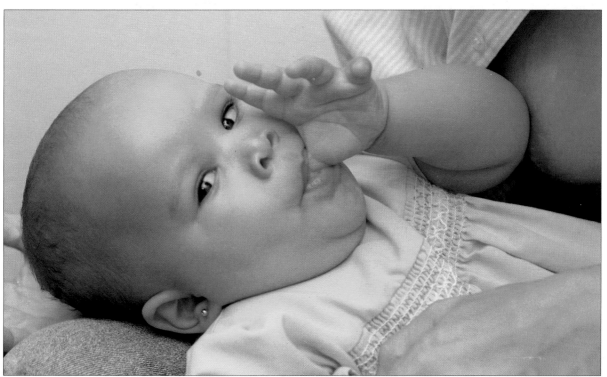

comforting, too – simply being held, stroked or patted, or hearing your voice or the voice of someone else she knows well. If you are sensitive to your baby's responses, you will know just when you can provide other forms of comfort. Until that time is reached – often during the second month of life – the breast is the surest remedy for a baby's distress. You are not conditioning her to have the nipple constantly in her mouth by offering that comfort readily and freely.

Playing with the nipple

When a baby is not hungry, but is luxuriating in the sweetness of the breast, she may play with and nibble the nipple. A baby often purses her lips and pushes the nipple out from the back of her mouth so that she is just getting the odd drip of milk – not the full flood that comes when she uses her jaw to pump milk from the breast. Interspersed with this nipple-nibbling, her mouth makes little twitching, smiling movements. She starts to suck again vigorously for a few seconds as if to tell you she is still busily occupied. But you know, and the baby knows, that the feeding has finished.

Sucking at one breast

Sometimes one breastful of milk is enough. A woman with a physical disability or who has a one-sided mastectomy can nurse at one side only. It is much better to continue at one breast until the baby indicates by her behavior that she has had enough, than to take her off and move her over to the other side because you believe you must use both breasts at each nursing.

If you constantly switch your baby from one breast to the other, the baby will get a large amount of dilute foremilk, but her hunger may never be satisfied. Foremilk is high in lactose. A baby who takes in too much lactose cannot break down and digest this form of sugar. Instead, gas is produced, which leads to a distended stomach, pockets of bubbles in the large intestine, jet-propelled bowel movements often flecked with green, pain, and long bouts of distressed crying.

Relieving a full breast

If you are left after nursing with one breast well used and the other feeling as if it is about to pop because it is so full, put a hot face cloth on the overloaded breast or squeeze warm water on it as you lean over a wash basin, and let the excess milk flow out. If you wish, you can express the milk and store it for later use (see pages 136–9).

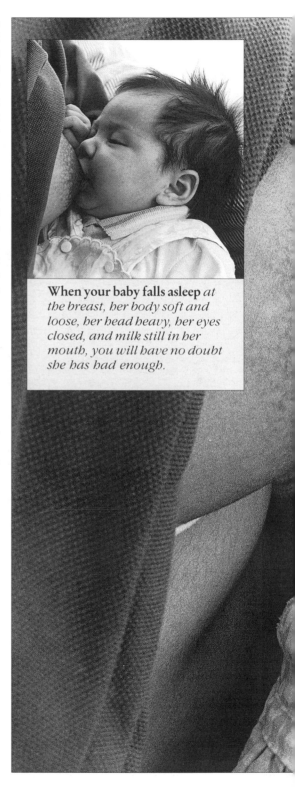

When your baby falls asleep *at the breast, her body soft and loose, her head heavy, her eyes closed, and milk still in her mouth, you will have no doubt she has had enough.*

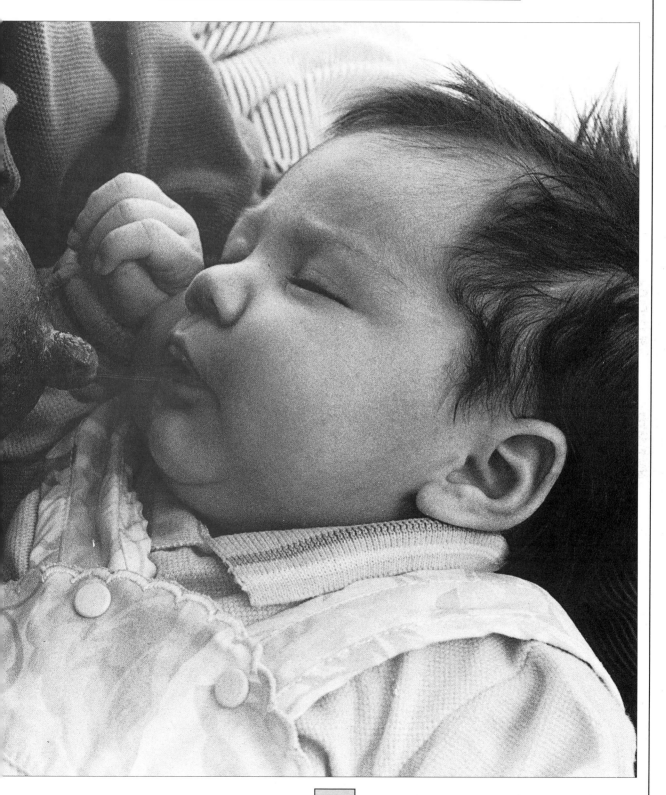

Sore & Cracked Nipples

SORE NIPPLES CAN DEVELOP CRACKS if not treated early. Cracked nipples can be agony. The main cause of sore nipples is poor positioning of the baby at the breast. A baby who is not latched on correctly tends to chew on the nipple stem in an attempt to obtain milk. (See pages 30–39 for the technique of latching on.)

Sometimes only one nipple becomes sore while the other one is all right. This is because it is simpler to latch the baby onto one breast rather than the other. If this is the case with you, try a different position when nursing your baby: hold her *under* your right arm, with her feet pointing behind. Then cradle her head in your hand, and let your breast drop into her mouth.

Another cause of sore nipples is using soap, creams, and lotions to which you are sensitive. Bubble baths, lanolin-based creams, and antiseptics sold to relieve nipple soreness may actually cause it or exacerbate the soreness.

Mouth infection
A yeast infection in your baby's mouth can also result in nipple soreness. Candida (thrush) consists of small white areas in the mouth which cannot be shifted when you touch them with your finger. The baby's mouth gets sore as well as your nipple, and you will continue to reinfect each other unless you are both treated.

One form of treatment is to apply the medication prescribed by your doctor or pediatrician to your baby's mouth immediately before nursing, so that when the baby latches onto the breast your nipples receive the benefit as well.

Treating sore nipples
Always offer your baby the least tender breast first. It will also help if you nurse your baby before she is desperately hungry, so that her sucking is less vigorous. Allow her to suck her fill on the first breast before putting her on the other breast, if she wants it, for as long as she

likes. If she has sucked well at the first breast, she may need very little from the other side, or not want it at all, so that the tender nipple can rest and recover.

Sore nipples heal quickly in the air, so if you get the chance to walk around topless, this will help. At night sleep naked, and lie on a towel to soak up any leaking milk. Avoid using plastic-lined bra pads as they trap moisture. When you get dressed, you might want to use breast shields (which are different from nipple shields). These can be obtained from lactation consultants. Breast shields help air to circulate around your breasts.

Some women find that smoothing in a little breastmilk over the tender area at the end of a feeding helps healing. They let their nipples dry in the warm air from a hair dryer or a light bulb. Others prefer to pat their nipples dry and then smooth on a lotion, calendula cream, or Vitamin E oil. Experiment to find out what is right for you.

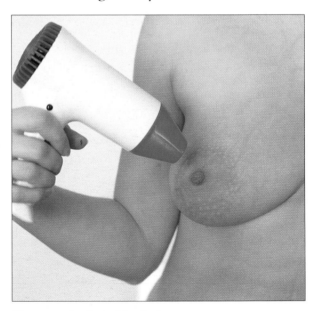

Dry sore nipples with a hair dryer *set on a gentle heat* (above) *after each feeding. This will soothe them and the warm air will help them heal.*

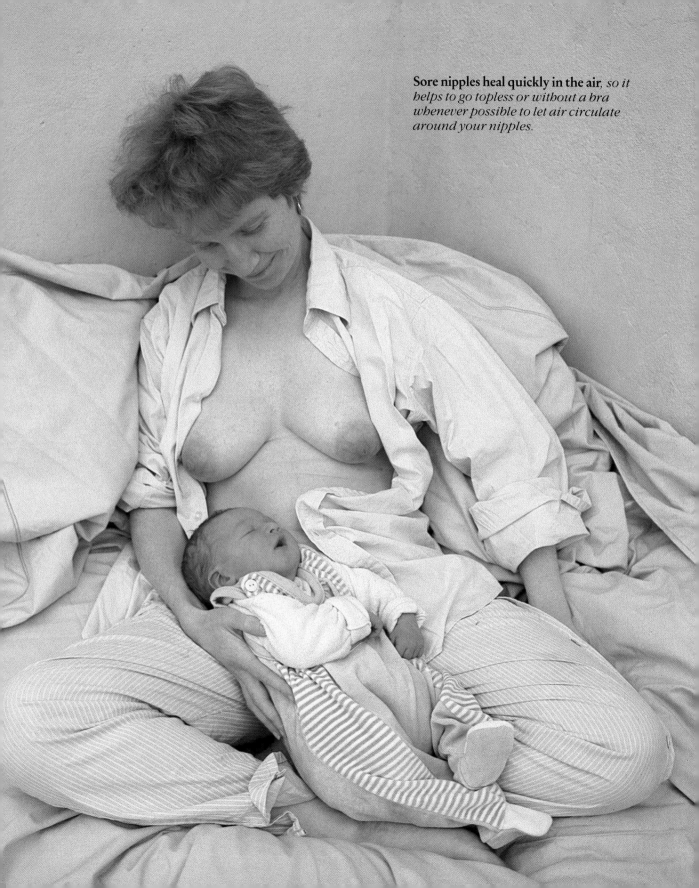

Sore nipples heal quickly in the air, *so it helps to go topless or without a bra whenever possible to let air circulate around your nipples.*

Engorgement & Mastitis

Engorged breasts are distended – sometimes so much so that the nipple retreats under surrounding tissue. They feel like hot bricks, and are extremely painful to touch. If not treated rapidly, engorgement will lead to mastitis, which is congestion of the milk ducts and inflammation of the breast.

What causes engorgement?

Engorgement is preventable. It is caused either by imposing long intervals between feedings – especially overnight – so that the breasts are not sufficiently emptied, or by bad positioning of the baby at the breast so that milk is not adequately drained from the lactiferous sinuses. If you are a copious milk producer, even one hurried nursing in which the baby has not been well positioned, or an unusually long interval between feedings

because your baby is sleeping extra soundly, may lead to engorgement. The sooner you start treatment the better.

Treatment

To treat engorged breasts, sit in a hot bath or under a shower and express enough milk to make you feel comfortable again. (See pages 136–9 on methods of expressing milk.) Directing a hand-held spray of hot water on the breasts gives blessed relief. Once you are more comfortable, put the baby to the breast and nurse whenever she rouses.

To prevent your breasts from becoming engorged when you are apart from your baby at any time, express some milk as soon as you feel full. Express just enough to make you feel comfortable, or it will stimulate production of yet more milk.

AN ENGORGED BREAST

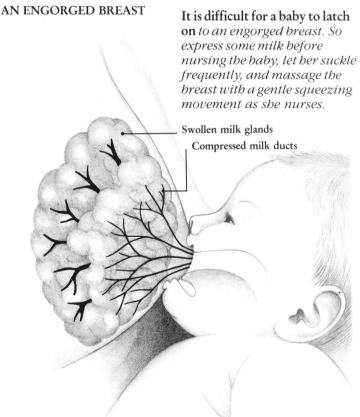

It is difficult for a baby to latch on *to an engorged breast. So express some milk before nursing the baby, let her suckle frequently, and massage the breast with a gentle squeezing movement as she nurses.*

Swollen milk glands
Compressed milk ducts

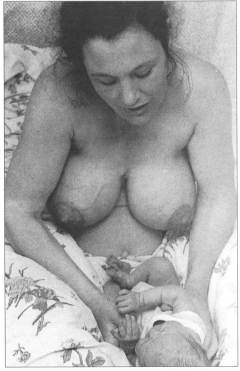

Engorged breasts are swollen, *hot, and tender. The milk-producing glands feel hard and lumpy, often under the arms.*

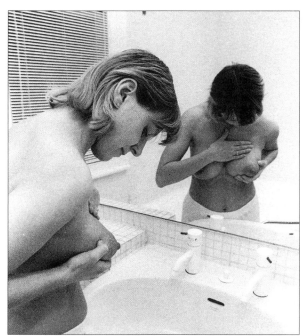

Expressing milk will help *to relieve an engorged breast. Lean over a wash basin to allow the milk to drip out, and gently massage the breast to encourage the milk to flow.*

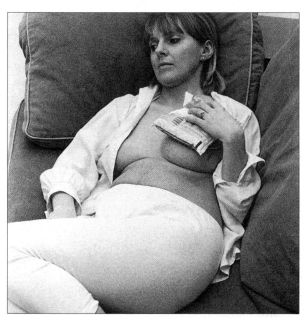

A packet of frozen peas *or a bag of ice-chips rested against a hot, engorged breast can feel very comforting and bring immediate relief.*

An engorged breast needs to be handled with great care. The swollen glands can easily be bruised. You may find that gently massaging your breasts will help to start the milk flowing but exercise extreme caution. It is safer for you to massage your breasts yourself than let anyone else do it for you.

MASTITIS

Mastitis is inflammation of the breast. A red area, which is tender to the touch, appears, often in the lower part of the right breast, and you develop a headache and run a temperature of 100°F or more. You feel feverish, tired, and aching.

The cause of mastitis is a blockage of milk in the ducts deep in the breast. It often occurs in the right breast in right-handed women because it is slightly more difficult to latch the baby on to the breast using the left hand. And it occurs more in the lower part because when you sit hunched up, this part of the breast is trapped against your body, and milk is not emptied from it. Wearing a bra that is too tight and which clasps the lower part of the breast against your body, or always holding the baby tensely, with your elbows firmly pressed against your breast, can have the same effect of trapping milk.

Treatment

The best way to treat mastitis is exactly the same as the best way to avoid it: ensure that the baby is correctly latched on so that she can empty the breast thoroughly.

If a red area develops, make certain that the baby's lower jaw clasps the part of the breast above where the inflammation has appeared. You can probably do this more easily if you tuck the baby's body under your arm with her feet pointing behind you, and cup her head in your hand to guide her into the right position. Alternatively, lie on your side with the baby lying alongside. Put the baby to the inflamed breast first. Lift your breast as you fix the baby on so that the lower part is not pressing against your ribcage.

Nurse as much as you can on the inflamed

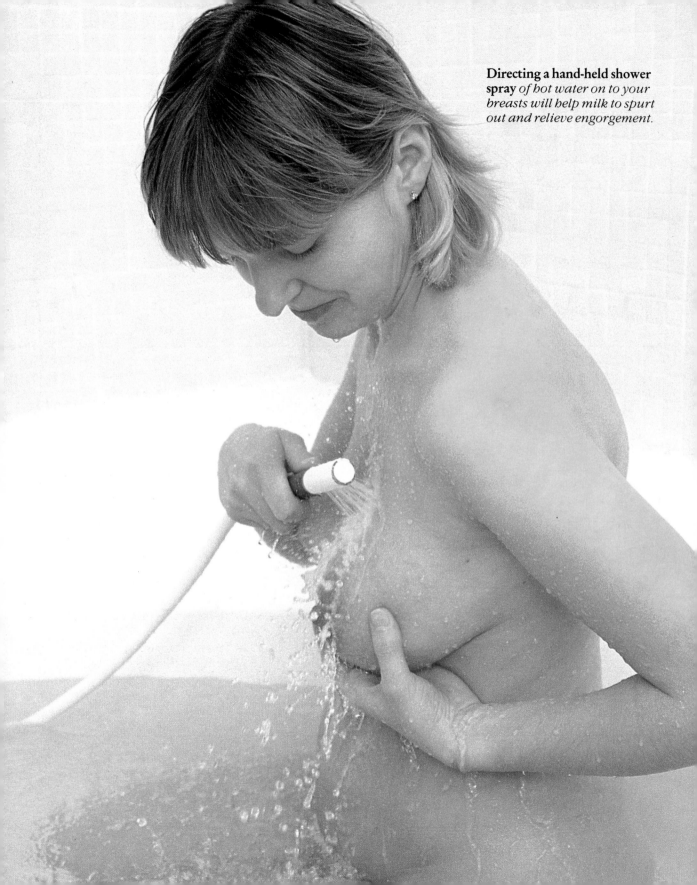

Directing a hand-held shower spray *of hot water on to your breasts will help milk to spurt out and relieve engorgement.*

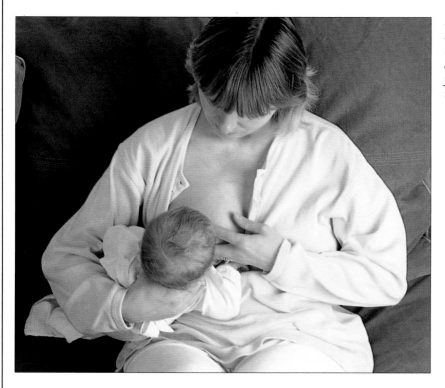

A good nursing position *if you have sore breasts is to tuck the baby's head under your arm, and cradle his head in your hand to direct his mouth right on to the "target area."*

side, the aim being to empty the breast of all the milk available. Some women use a breast pump to help them achieve this. The milk is perfectly safe for your baby, so do not throw it away – freeze it for a future time. A well-used breast does not get mastitis, so make sure that this breast is used thoroughly.

Before the baby comes to the breast, and during intervals in sucking, massage the sore part by pressing and squeezing it with your fingers deep in the glandular tissue. This will help free the milk.

Easing the discomfort

For your comfort, you can sponge your breast with warm water. Have frequent baths or showers, and either direct a spray of hot water on your breast, or kneel in the bath so that your breasts hang down into the warm water. When you are lying down or sitting and relaxing, you can rest a hot compress against the red area. Or you may prefer a cold one, the simplest and easiest being a small bag of frozen peas.

Do not forget your other breast while you are doing this. If the baby is not using the second breast as much, apply hot compresses and express milk to keep it flowing.

Any exercise that entails hitting a ball with an over-arm movement, such as tennis or badminton, is helpful as it increases blood circulation to the inflamed area and aids healing. Vigorous arm movements of the kind used in washing and wringing out cloths by hand will also help – something you may not usually want to do!

However, this does not mean that you should take on all the housework – you will benefit from as much sleep as you can get. If the mastitis is being relieved, your temperature will go down over a period of forty-eight hours, until it is normal again. But you will start to feel better, and the breast will feel softer and emptier, long before this. If you find self-treatment ineffective, see your doctor who will probably prescribe an antibiotic. Any antibiotic that can safely be given to an infant can be used by a nursing mother.

Getting Enough Sleep

It goes without saying that a new baby can be exhausting. Newborn babies do not know the difference between day and night, so they may fuss and want frequent feeding and attention at nighttime and sleep solidly during the morning or afternoon.

You will find yourself getting very tired if you go to bed at your usual hour and carry on during the day as if nothing has happened. You need to take every opportunity you can to rest during the twenty-four hours, even if it is at odd times. You may not want to sleep, but at least you can put your feet up and take it easy for half an hour.

Feeding at night

If your baby does not drop off to sleep right after a night feeding, your partner can scoop her up and take her to a different room to settle her down, so that you can sleep undisturbed. Then they can both creep back in without waking you, or bed down elsewhere, to make sure that you get a spell of uninterrupted sleep to restore your energy.

If you are adept at expressing milk, someone else may be able to feed the baby with a bottle of your milk at night. Though she may only sleep for an hour or so longer, and then want you – and only you – that extra time can give you some much needed rest.

Resting during the day

The time to catch up on extra sleep is immediately after your baby has nursed. If you leave it and do urgent work first, you may never get the chance. Look at the pattern of your baby's sleeping and waking and you can probably discover a time when she takes a longish nap.

If you have older children, you can still relax by setting aside a regular quiet time in the day with them, when you can read them a story, sing nursery rhymes, or do something peaceful like making cut-out dolls from a newspaper. You can also keep special playthings for this time, so that it is marked off from the rest of the day. The children will look forward to this time, too, because it is a space in the day for them, when they can have your full attention.

A new baby makes a lot of work – especially laundry. Use disposable diapers when you can and dress the baby in clothes that are easily washed and dried. If there is a chance of help with the chores, grasp it. It is more important that you get enough sleep, than catch up with other work.

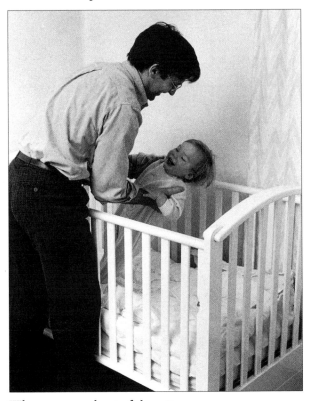

When you are short of sleep *it helps if someone else can take over responsibility for a while. If you express some milk, your partner can pick up the baby when he cries and give a bottle of breast-milk. As well as enabling you to catch up on your sleep, this lets your partner become more fully involved in caring for the baby.*

If You Are Ill

If you are ill while you are breastfeeding, it is more help to arrange for someone else to do the housework than for you to give up breast-feeding or hand over the care of the baby. Breastfeeding can make life easier for you. You do not have to spend time sterilizing bottles and filling them with formula. Instead, you can cuddle up in bed with the baby and enjoy each other. Knowing you can offer your milk increases your self-esteem and confidence as a mother at a time when you may be especially anxious.

The rush of prolactin and other hormones released into a woman's bloodstream while she is breastfeeding sometimes results in remission in symptoms of chronic illness. This applies particularly to diabetic mothers and those suffering from arthritis, lupus, and, possibly, multiple sclerosis.

If you are diabetic you may wonder whether your milk is safe for your baby. It is. Some studies show that breastfed babies develop diabetes less often.

Going to the hospital

If you have to go into the hospital, you should be able to take your baby in with you so that you can nurse her. If you have a general anes-thetic the drug will pass into your milk, so the baby should be given either your own or another mother's expressed milk in a bottle for twelve to twenty-four hours. When you are feeling weak or drowsy, someone else should be present to lift and change the baby.

Relactating

If you lose your milk when you are ill, you may decide you want to relactate. Your milk will return, but it will take up to ten days. You need to organize practical help so that you can lie in bed with your baby, letting her suck as much as she wants. This sucking is the most effective way of producing milk.

Empty your breasts with an electric pump four or five times a day after the baby has sucked. You can express this milk straight into a bottle and give it to her. At first you will only produce a few drops, but that is still a triumph. Bottle-feed the baby after she has had some time at the breast, but as you feel your own milk return, gradually reduce this.

Taking drugs when breastfeeding

If you can, avoid all drugs when breast-feeding. When you *have* to take medicine there are usually drugs available which only have a slight effect on the baby. The most usual effect is to make the baby rather drowsy (tranquilizers and antihistamines) or the stools very loose (antibiotics).

ORAL CONTRACEPTIVES Birth control pills may reduce your milk supply *when you first take them*. Nurse more frequently to build up the supply again. The combined estrogen-proges-terone pill should not be taken when you are breastfeeding.

ANTIBIOTICS Avoid chloramphenicol, since 50 per cent of the dose appears in breastmilk. Flagyl, often prescribed for urinary infections, passes into milk in large quantities, too. Nali-dixic should not be taken as it may produce anemia in the baby. Other antibiotics are all right. When you are taking antibiotics you may find that your baby is especially thirsty.

SEDATIVES These slow down metabolism, and so reduce the production of breastmilk. In order to stimulate the supply, the baby will need feeding more often.

If you need to take Valium you can reckon that only 10 per cent of the amount in your own circulation passes through the milk into the baby. But it is best to avoid it in the first weeks of your baby's life as it can build up and cause reduced muscle tone. An older baby can get rid of Valium more efficiently.

ANTI-DEPRESSANTS These probably have little effect on a baby, and nortriptyline has not been found in breastmilk. Fifty per cent of lithium passes into breastmilk in the first week of life, but after that time the baby excretes it more effectively, and only about one-third appears in the baby's blood. Reduced muscle tone and poor circulation are two signs that will tell you that a baby is receiving too high a dose of lithium in the milk.

LAXATIVES The type that adds bulk to feces is not absorbed from your intestinal tract. They are better for the baby than purgatives which make your bowels work faster and may make the baby's stools loose.

DRUGS FOR EPILEPSY Phenytoin is safe for a baby. Though 50 per cent of the drug in the mother's circulation passes into the breast-milk, the baby is able to excrete it readily. Carbamazepine passes into breastmilk in a higher concentration – about 60 per cent – but does not seem to harm the baby.

DIURETICS These should not be taken because they reduce the milk supply.

DRUGS FOR LOW BLOOD PRESSURE Drugs to raise blood pressure are excreted in breastmilk, but no side effects have been observed.

DRUGS FOR ASTHMA Some drugs taken for asthma can make the baby fretful. If you have to take theophylline, avoid coffee, tea, and chocolate – all of which contain caffeine – as when taken in combination they tend to have a cumulative effect.

STEROIDS A woman who is prescribed steroids to treat asthma, rheumatoid arthritis, or cancer, is usually advised not to breastfeed. Steroids taken in the form of an inhaler do not affect the baby. Systemic steroids, taken by mouth, pass into the bloodstream and into your milk. If you are prescribed systemic steroids for a period of not longer than ten days, express and freeze what milk you can before taking the first dose.

RADIOACTIVE IODINE This will affect the baby's thyroid gland, so you should not breastfeed while taking it. Express milk and store it in advance in the refrigerator or freezer. Express milk to keep the supply going and throw it away until twelve hours after you have stopped taking the radioactive iodine.

ANTI-COAGULANTS Most anti-coagulants are not dangerous for babies. Coumadin and heparin are passed into milk. Dicumarol has not been found to change blood clotting time in breast-fed babies.

"I've never felt as tired as this in my life. You're a very unreasonable baby. You treat me like a milk dispenser that has to be on tap day and night – but I love you!"

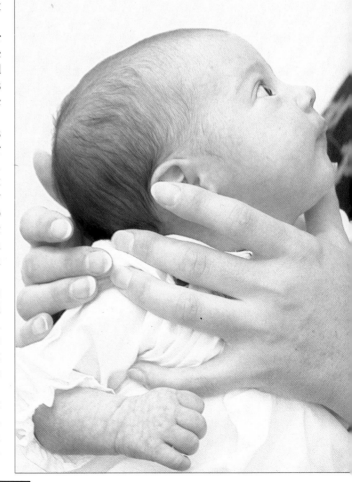

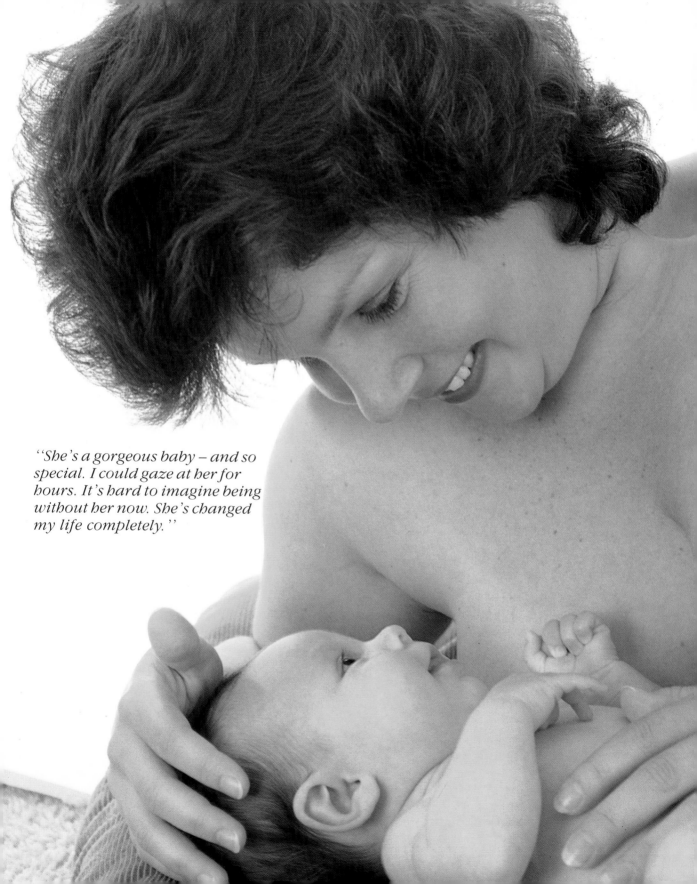

''She's a gorgeous baby – and so special. I could gaze at her for hours. It's hard to imagine being without her now. She's changed my life completely.''

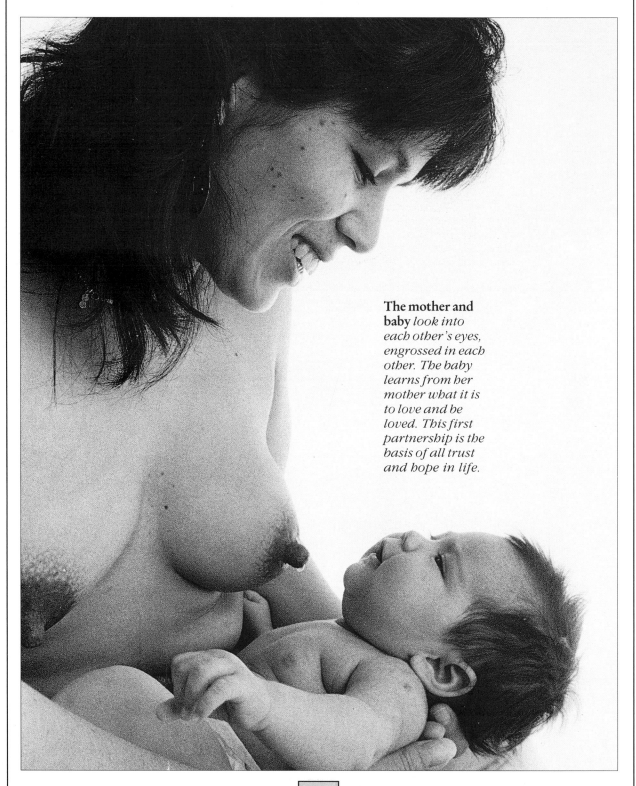

The mother and baby *look into each other's eyes, engrossed in each other. The baby learns from her mother what it is to love and be loved. This first partnership is the basis of all trust and hope in life.*

TRYING TO FOCUS

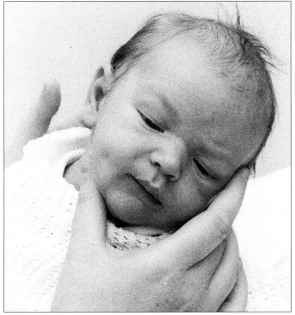

1 *When you hold your baby and look into his face, he may at first appear uninterested in you and look away.*

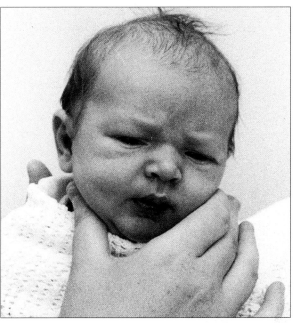

2 *He will scan his field of vision, actively looking for something interesting. At first both eyes cannot coordinate easily.*

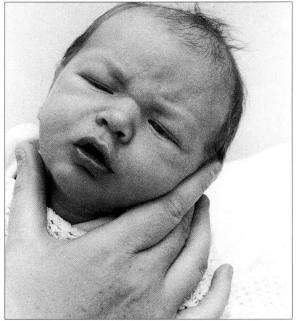

3 *Then he catches sight of you and squints as he tries to focus, for what he can see is fuzzy and blurred at the edges.*

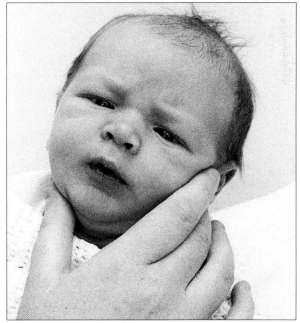

4 *After some trial and error, he gazes at you with concentration and a slight frown as if to say, "Is this really my mother?"*

The Sleepy Baby

Some babies need to be encouraged to latch on and suck at the breast because they are sleepy. Premature babies are often like this. A baby who is too hot may also be hard to rouse. Some very sleepy babies are, in fact, underfed babies who are dehydrated and who have reduced muscle tone. Some babies may also be drowsy in the days following birth because of anesthetics they have received during labor.

Once you enable a baby to draw in a good mouthful of breast so that the milk flows copiously, his whole character often changes. A passive, sleepy baby becomes wide-awake and interested in his surroundings. After a few satisfying feedings like this, his muscle tone improves dramatically, you see a bloom and freshness on his skin, his eyes shine, and he takes each feeding with gusto. Your relationship with the baby then becomes livelier and more rewarding.

Stimulating the baby to nurse

There are several things you can do to stimulate a sleepy baby to take the breast. First, and most important, make sure that your baby is positioned against you correctly (see pages 30–39 on latching on). If your breast is distended, express some milk before nursing to make it easier for the baby to latch on.

Tease the baby with the breast by squeezing out a few drops of milk so that he can smell and perhaps lick it. Talk to, stroke, and woo him. Make him more alert by partially undressing him so that his feet are cool. This wakes up some babies immediately. Turn off bright lights and nurse the baby in half-light. Babies open their eyes and become more interested in their surroundings when the light is not glaring.

If your milk ejection reflex is slow to come and the baby loses interest before you feel the tingling, buzzing sensation in the other breast, apply a warm towel or face cloth to your breasts before nursing. If you feel very anxious, try using some of the childbirth breathing exercises or other relaxation techniques to help the milk start to flow.

Occasionally, a baby who has already become accustomed to a bottle may manage more easily at the breast if you use a latex nipple shield over your nipple. Once he is sucking well, and has paused for a moment, you may be able to slip the nipple shield off and get him latched on to your breast.

A baby who is often only half awake, *and not at all sure that he wants to nurse, may have to be given some encouragement.*

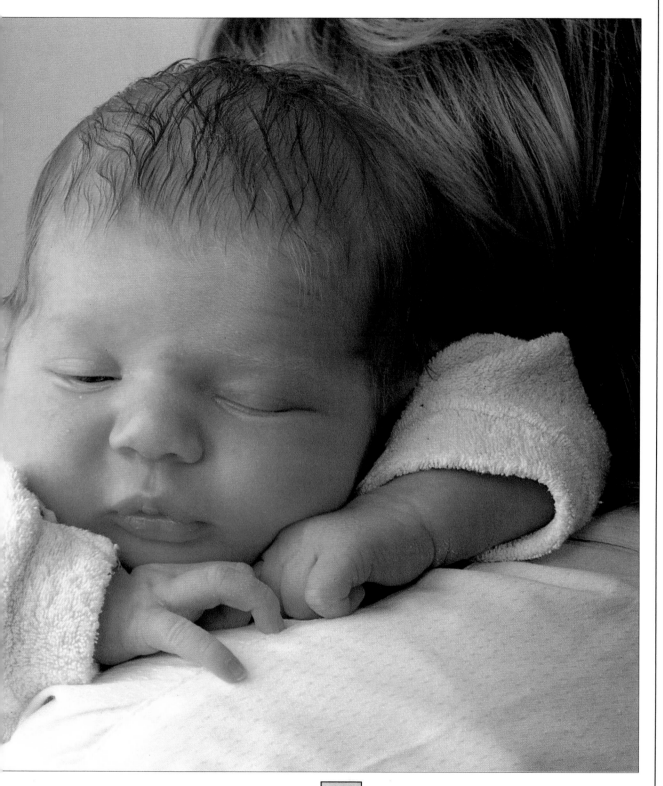

ENCOURAGING A BABY TO NURSE

1 *Talk to your baby. Show him things that shine or move. See if you can make eye contact. Stroke his head, and trace the lines of his nose, eyebrows, ears, and mouth with your fingers, talking to him all the time.*

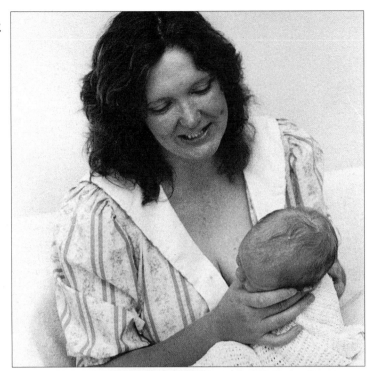

2 *Squeeze out a little milk so that it glistens like a pearl on the surface of your nipple. Tantalize your baby with it. When he smells how delicious it is, he may become interested enough to suck.*

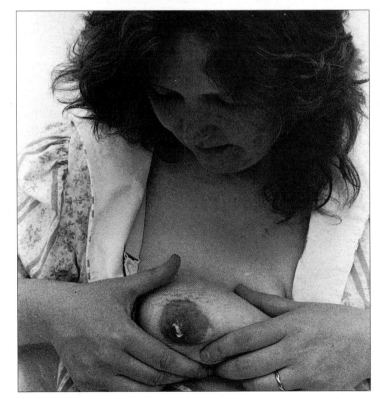

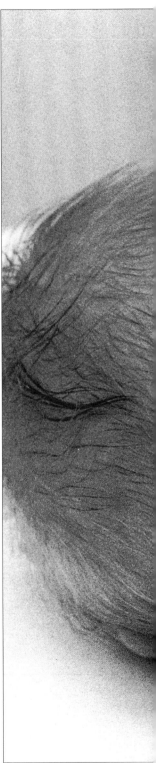

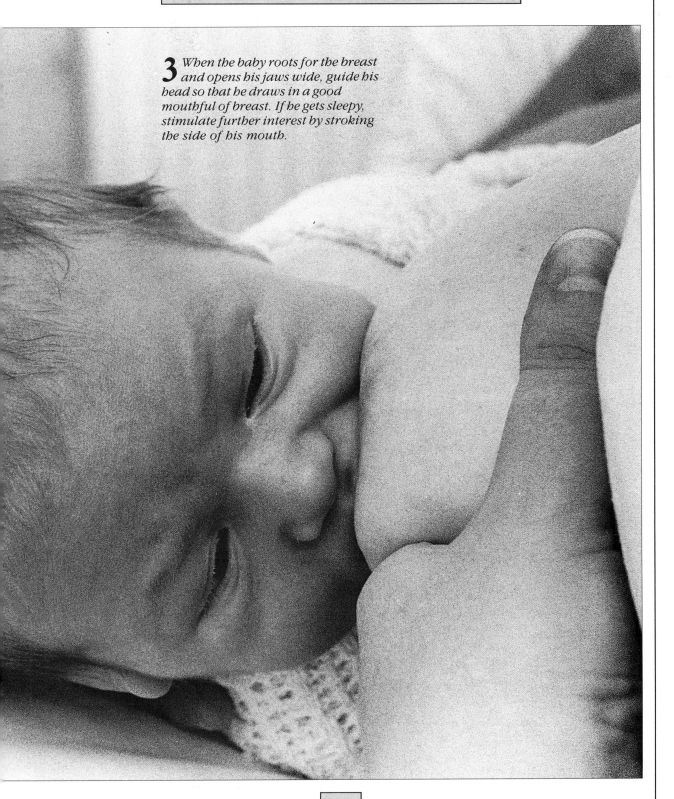

3 *When the baby roots for the breast and opens his jaws wide, guide his head so that he draws in a good mouthful of breast. If he gets sleepy, stimulate further interest by stroking the side of his mouth.*

The Excited Baby

An excited baby may need to be calmed down before she will take the breast. If your baby cries furiously for food, but then resists being put to the breast, arching her back, pummeling you with her fists and turning purple with rage, don't struggle with her. Do something quite different, such as changing her diaper, or putting her over your shoulder and patting her bottom, until she has quieted down a bit. Or hand her to someone else for a few minutes – when in your arms she is stimulated and aroused by your own body scent, the smell of your milk, and the nearness of your breasts.

Soothing a fretful baby

A baby who is restless and fretful, but not actually screaming, often quiets if you rest your head against hers and hum a resonant tune or just a few deep, melodious sounds. As soon as she is contented, offer the breast gently but quickly.

Babies who are very easily stimulated often like to nurse in a room with only dim light, or with their eyes protected by a shawl, and they sometimes like a background of soothing music. If your baby is like this, see if you can go to a quiet room away from other people so that your baby can nurse peacefully. Some babies get so angry in their first weeks, and seem so frightened by their anger, that they are happiest when cocooned firmly in a big towel or blanket with only the head visible.

Babies undergo all sorts of uncomfortable experiences, many of which are unavoidable since they are connected with internal sensations and with the baby's adjustment to life. A baby who is bombarded by stimuli from inside cannot really concentrate on the outside world and on the things you are doing to help her. But one of the most important things you can do for your baby – from birth onward – is to reach out to comfort her as soon as she becomes distressed. You won't always manage to soothe her. But at least she will know you are trying and so will you.

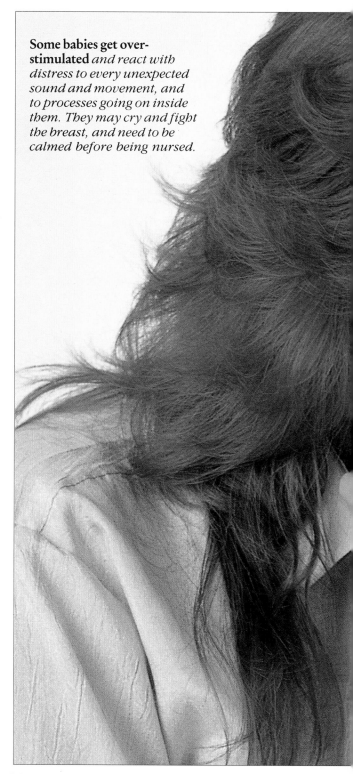

Some babies get over-stimulated *and react with distress to every unexpected sound and movement, and to processes going on inside them. They may cry and fight the breast, and need to be calmed before being nursed.*

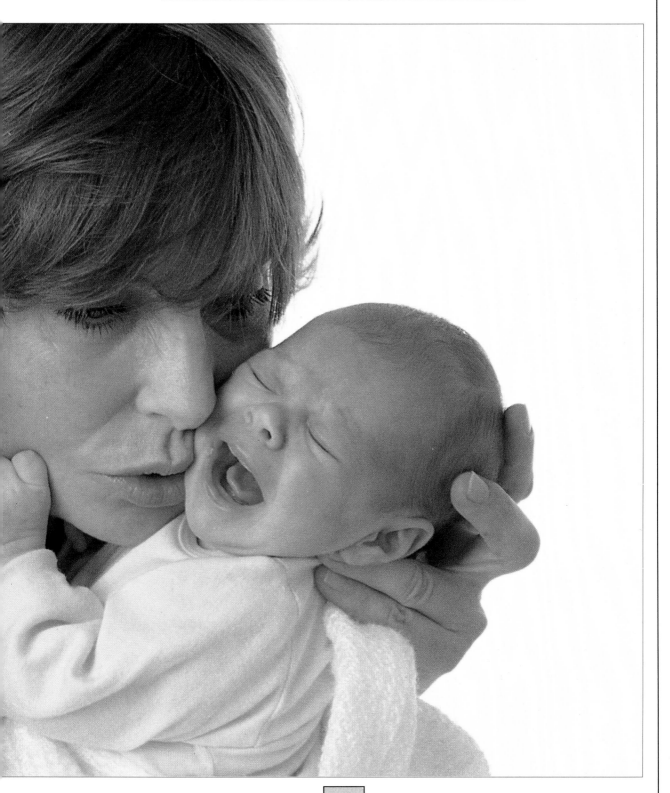

WRAPPING AN EXCITED BABY

1 *An over-excited newborn baby may calm down eventually if wrapped in a large, soft shawl, towel, or receiving blanket. Here an experienced midwife places the baby on a big shawl on her lap and begins to wrap him up. She talks soothingly as she does so, telling him what a beautiful baby he is.*

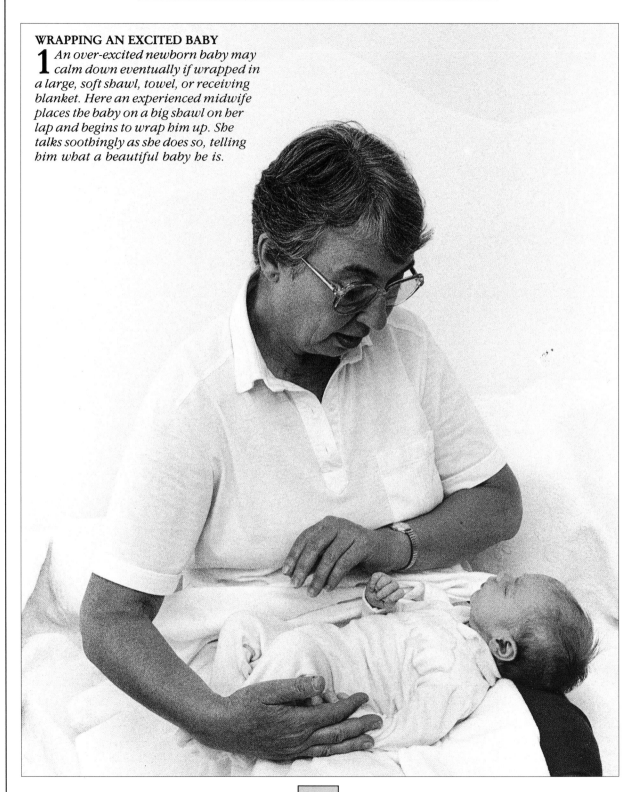

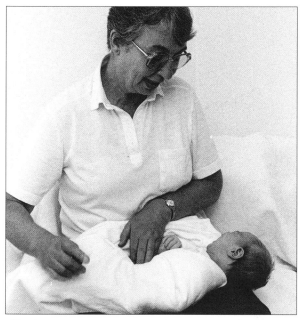

2 *She draws up one side of the shawl, and tucks it tightly around the baby, moving slowly and deliberately, and talking softly all the time.*

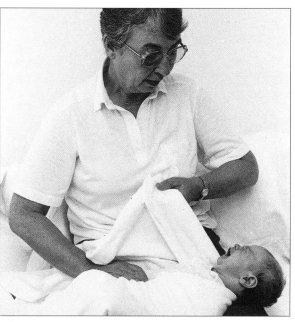

3 *Then she brings up the other side of the shawl, quietly and confidently, and tucks the baby's arms firmly against his body.*

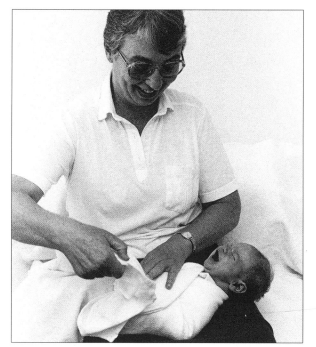

4 *She makes a solid, tight bundle, so that the shawl holds the baby rather as the muscles of the uterus must have grasped him before birth.*

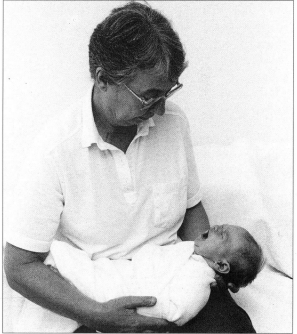

5 *It didn't work! The baby is still angry, though now she has him encased from neck to toes as neatly as a pea in a pod!*

Digestive Adventures

Babies are often overwhelmed by their digestive processes and all the alarming things that are going on inside them.

Adapting to the outside world

Before birth the baby is fed automatically from your bloodstream, the nutritious elements percolating through the placenta directly into his bloodstream. Not only does he not have to do any work to get food, but it is instantly available, without even a half-second pause. In fact, it flows continuously into his body. So it must feel very odd to your newborn baby to have things squeezing and bumping, opening, and constricting inside him when he is not used to it.

As milk goes down the esophagus, it is helped toward the stomach by regular muscular tightening of the tube. The milk residue enters the intestines and is directed down to the colon in the same way. All these actions often become unsynchronized, especially if the baby has been gulping hungrily or crying furiously. Sometimes it seems to happen if the mother has eaten foods to which the baby is not yet accustomed. All these new digestive adventures your baby is experiencing are clearly visible to you – he may screw up his face in surprise, frown, squirm, writhe, and become miserable.

Comforting your baby

A baby who is engrossed in a digestive experience like this is best held upright against your shoulder or laid down on his tummy on your lap. Pat him on the bottom with a slow, regular rhythm. Warmth may help – rest a covered hot water bottle a little higher than body heat, or a face cloth wrung out in hot water, against his tummy. But make sure that nothing is too hot as babies burn easily. Talk soothing nonsense words to him, or sing softly, so that the baby hears from the tone of your voice, and learns from your own confidence, that these internal events are not catastrophic and will soon pass.

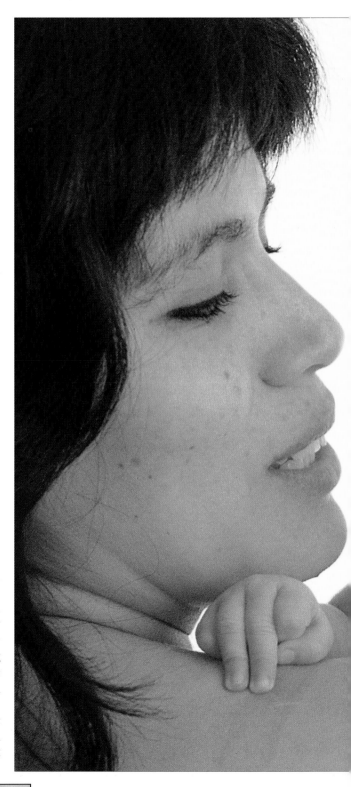

A baby may feel bombarded *by strange and unsettling sensations going on inside her during the process of digestion. She may feel uncomfortable and even frightened. Holding the baby upright over your shoulder or on your lap helps her feel safe and she will come to accept the extraordinary feelings.*

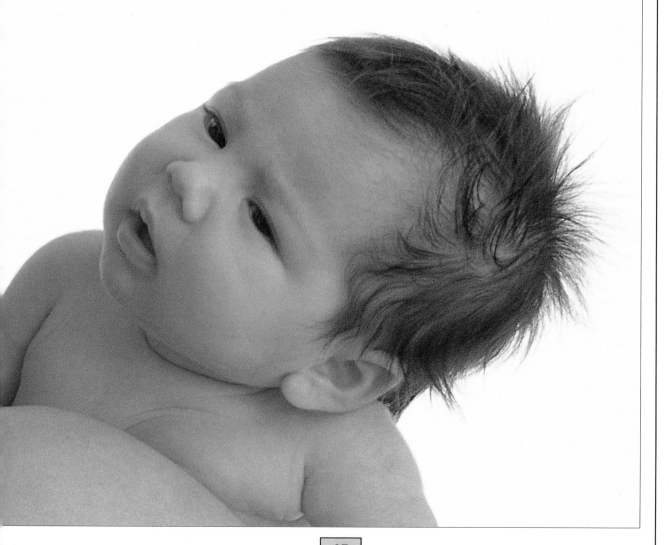

SOOTHING A BABY
Lie your baby on his tummy on your lap after nursing. He will be comforted by the warmth from your body as you pat or rub his back. Let your knees support the baby's chest and thighs, as a full tummy feels better if there is no pressure against it.

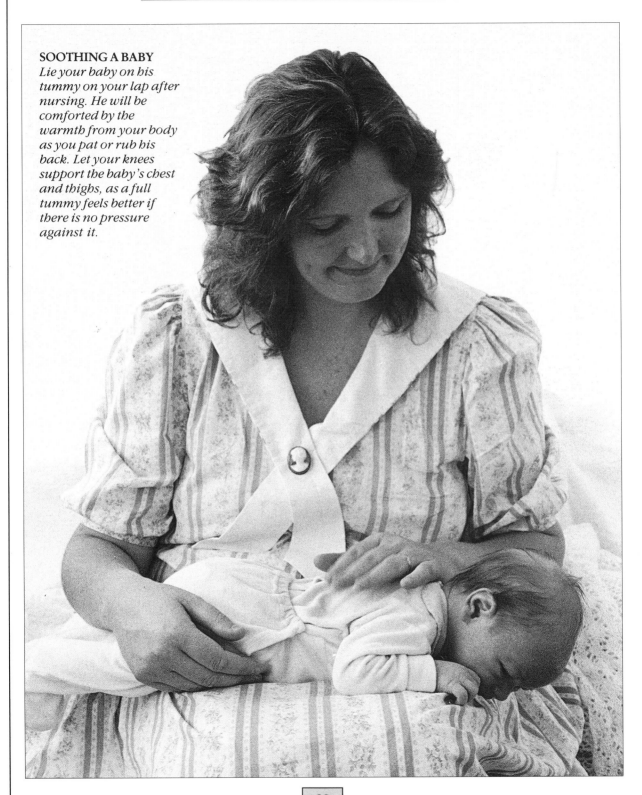

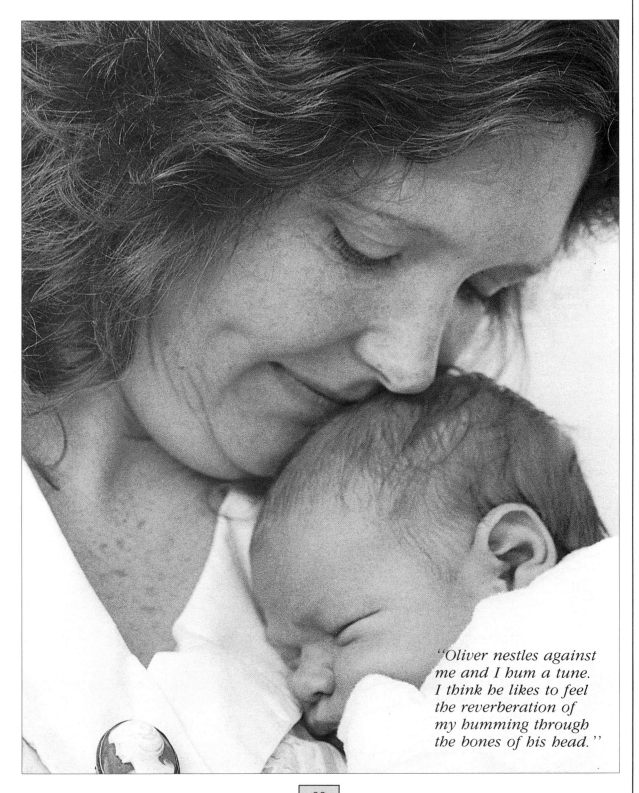

"Oliver nestles against
me and I hum a tune.
I think he likes to feel
the reverberation of
my humming through
the bones of his head."

Introducing Other Pleasures

You do not have to put the baby to the breast every time she cries. In the first two or three weeks of life, crying can probably only be assuaged by giving the breast, but after that the world opens out and new delights blossom. If all you ever offer your baby is the breast, you may find yourself going around with one hanging out for hours on end – just in case!

New experiences

When your baby is restless she may want something other than food – to be cuddled, for example, to float in warm water, to move to another position, or perhaps to kick on her back with no clothes on. Or she may like to have a soothing massage, listen to music or a tinkling bell, or watch a dancing mobile or shadows on the wall. Early on, your baby learns that there are other pleasures in life besides breastfeeding. If you can see when she is ready for a variety of new learning experiences, you will contribute to her development as an integrated human being who is secure in herself and who can use her environment for further learning.

Yet if you are very tired, you probably feel that nursing is just about all you can do, and that you haven't the time for anything else except laundry and basic housework. However, doing things with your baby, playing with her, watching her develop, receiving responses from her, and sometimes being rewarded with a smile or a chuckle – this makes the hard work and the broken nights worthwhile. So even if you are feeling over-tired, it is important for you both that you have time to enjoy each other.

Bath-time

Bathing your baby is one of those special activities which can be the high point of the day for you both. (In fact, there is no reason why a baby cannot have several baths a day.) Putting a baby in a warm, comforting bath is one of the best ways of breaking tension and helps her – and you – to relax. Until you are confident, test the water with a thermometer – it should be as warm as your baby's body (85°F). Ensure that the room is comfortably warm, too. Buy some big, soft bath towels you can pre-warm so that you can bundle her up cosily afterward. Never leave a baby in a bath unattended, however much she enjoys it, even though you are just on the other side of the door.

Some babies experience near ecstasy *in the bath. They can move freely, kick vigorously, and make exciting splashes, and the occasional tidal wave, all the time with an adoring audience. They soon learn to close their eyes to keep out the water. A baby may enjoy lying unsupported in shallow water, but never leave him alone.*

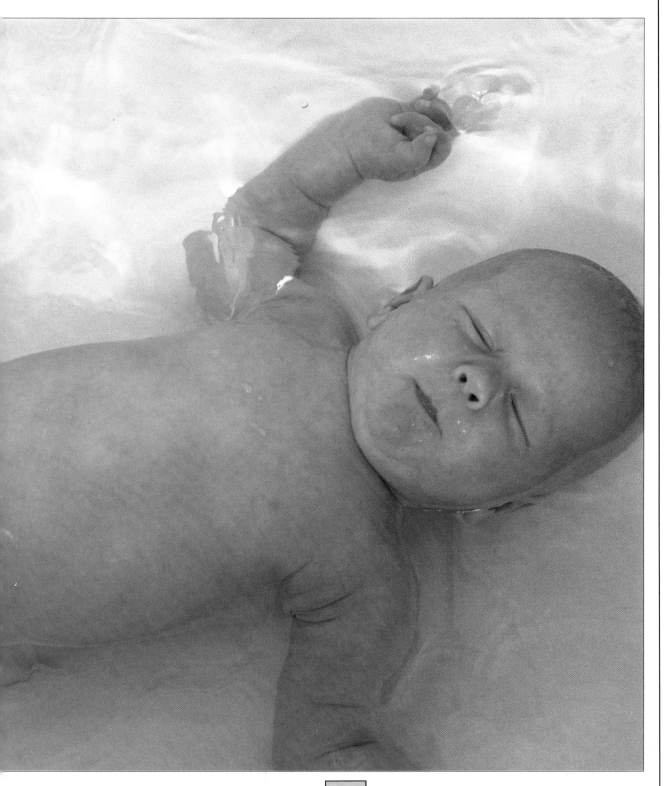

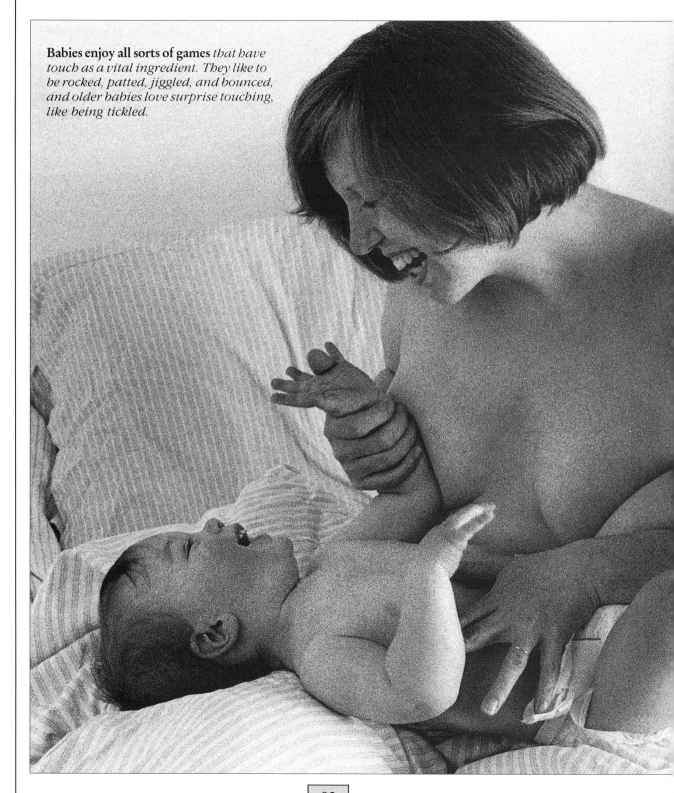

Babies enjoy all sorts of games *that have touch as a vital ingredient. They like to be rocked, patted, jiggled, and bounced, and older babies love surprise touching, like being tickled.*

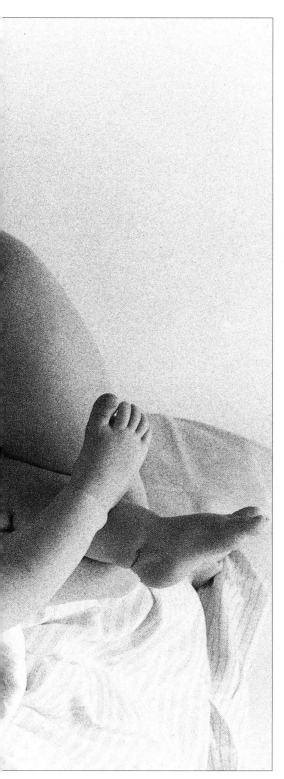

It is important to offer new experiences only when the baby is calm, happy, and responsive. Do not push things. Just wait and see what happens, and enjoy it when your baby eagerly reaches out to grasp these new and exciting experiences.

Stimulating the senses

Even when a baby is only a few days old, she will enjoy her senses being stimulated in different ways if in a quiet, alert state. She may like to smell a lemon, or freshly ground coffee, or herbs, garlic, or lavender from the garden. Present each smell separately and simply give the baby the opportunity to investigate and concentrate on experiencing it.

Long before you are thinking about introducing solid foods, your baby may like to smell and taste a variety of things: a grape, perhaps, or a peeled and pitted cherry. When you offer these things, do not put them in the baby's mouth – rest the object lightly against her lips and observe what happens. Even a baby of a few weeks old may like a few licks of a fruit popsicle if the weather is hot. But give plenty of time for the baby to savor and appreciate the taste and smell of the new experience you are presenting.

Looking and learning

Babies have strong visual preferences. They do not stare passively at anything and everything. They select what interests them. They enjoy the play of light and shadow on a wall. They gaze with concentrated pleasure at textured fabrics and intricate patterns. They prefer patterned to plain surfaces, even if the plain ones are brightly colored, and they like three-dimensional objects and things that move. You can show your baby swirls and zig-zags, stripes, squares, circles and diamonds – anything with a strong pattern. Patchwork is a never-failing source of delight. Babies also like to see lace and muslin move in the breeze, which is why cradles used to be hung with lace and frilly things.

Your baby is also busy learning: she watches people's eyes and mouths and hears the sounds they produce, she copies the shapes formed by their mouths, smiles, and receives a smile in return. She learns to anticipate other people's behavior – knowing that when bath water is running, something good is about to happen, that when she is put on her back in a certain way she is about to have a diaper changed, or that when lying on her tummy she is expected to go to sleep.

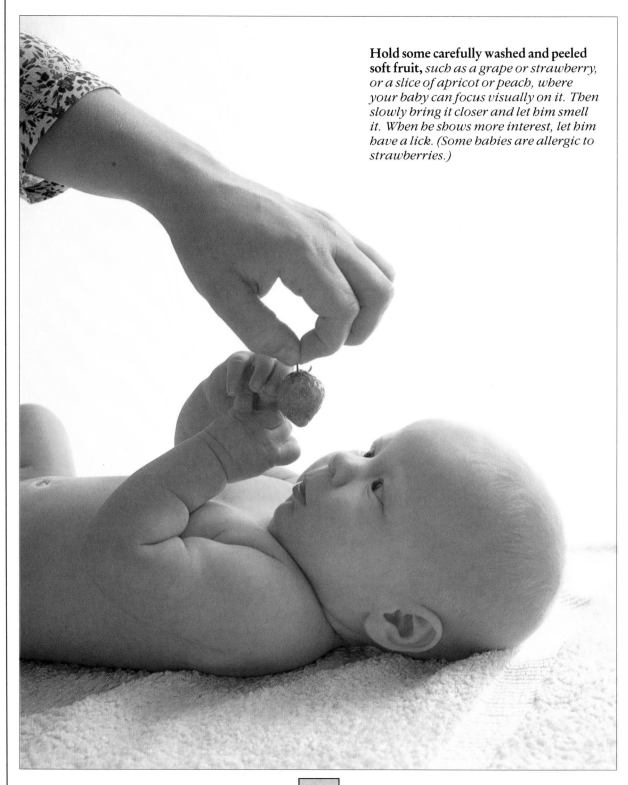

Hold some carefully washed and peeled soft fruit, *such as a grape or strawberry, or a slice of apricot or peach, where your baby can focus visually on it. Then slowly bring it closer and let him smell it. When he shows more interest, let him have a lick. (Some babies are allergic to strawberries.)*

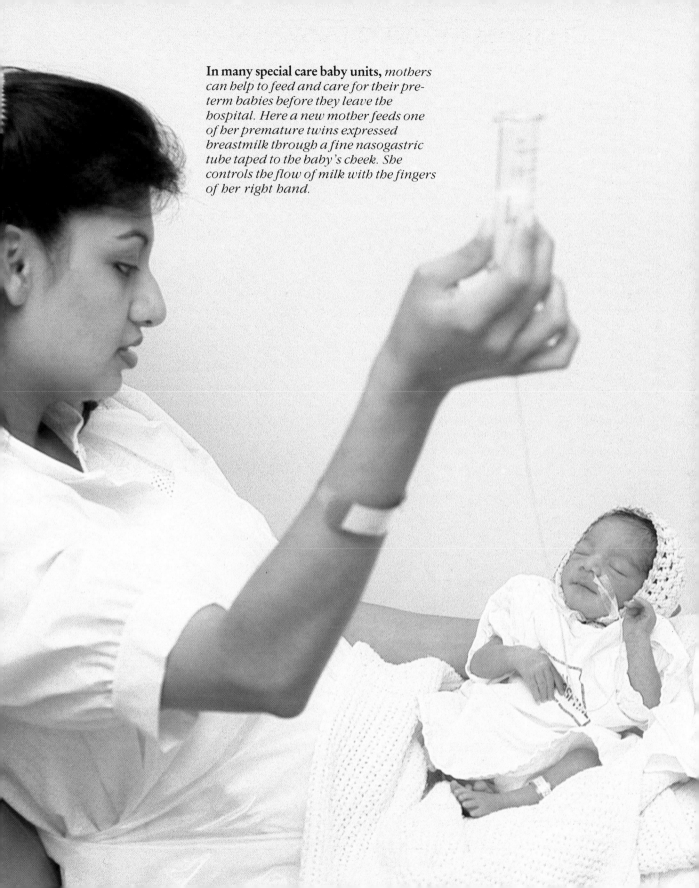

In many special care baby units, *mothers can help to feed and care for their pre-term babies before they leave the hospital. Here a new mother feeds one of her premature twins expressed breastmilk through a fine nasogastric tube taped to the baby's cheek. She controls the flow of milk with the fingers of her right hand.*

When your baby is ready to suck, it will probably only be for a very short time at first, as she gets tired quickly. So you begin a feeding by putting her to the breast, and then, when she is finding it hard work, perhaps add expressed milk, and finish – if necessary – by tube feeding. Though it is exciting to know that the baby is sucking at last, it is a very slow process, and you may feel depressed and very tired yourself.

A pre-term or ill baby may have to be taught how to latch on to the breast correctly and even how to suck (see pages 30-39). To help stimulate the correct movement of the jaw when your baby is getting weary, put a finger under her chin and exert gentle pressure.

Your baby will be test-weighed at each feeding to see how much she taking and to determine whether your milk needs supplementing. Some pediatricians supplement all pre-term babies, however much milk their mothers produce, and you may want to discuss this with your pediatrician.

You will need to find out exactly what your baby's feeding schedule is, so that you can be in the nursery at the right times to put her to the breast. It can be very upsetting to arrive there only to find that the baby has been fed, is now asleep, and you are dismissed.

Even when your baby is sucking well at the breast, continue to use the pump at the end of each nursing, as this will stimulate your milk supply. Go on doing this until breastfeeding is well established and you feel confident.

Going home

Then there comes the time when you are able to take your baby home.

Ask the hospital to keep frozen any of your expressed breastmilk that remains, as it may come in useful when you get home. If your baby gets tired at the breast, for example, you can finish with a bottle of your own milk. Bottle-feeding often demands less effort from the baby than breastfeeding. Sometimes it takes a few weeks before your baby can suck sufficiently strongly to satisfy her appetite fully at the breast.

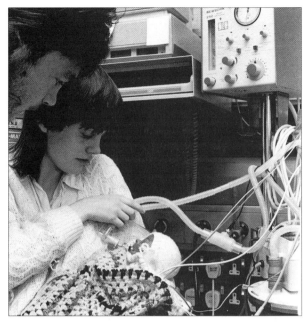

Feeding your premature baby yourself, *while she is in the high tech setting of a special care unit, helps you feel that she belongs to you.*

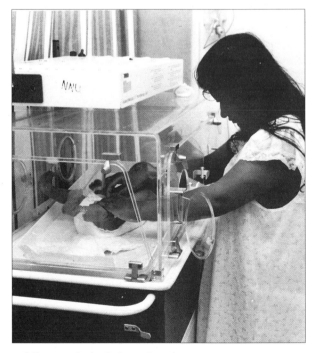

While your baby is in an incubator, *you can change her diaper and gently stroke and massage her through the port-holes.*

The Jaundiced Baby

If your three- or four-day-old baby looks as if she has just come back from a holiday in the tropics and is beautifully tanned, the chances are that she has jaundice. Four or five babies in every ten develop some yellowing of the eyes and skin – especially the legs – at this time, which gradually fades until it disappears entirely when they are a week or two old.

Causes of jaundice

Most of these babies are completely healthy. This "physiological" jaundice occurs because of the breakdown of red cells in the baby's blood. While in the uterus the baby has a higher proportion of red blood cells than it needs after birth. This enables her to get good oxygenation inside your body.

During pregnancy the placenta filters out waste products from the red blood cells. Once the baby is born her own liver must break down this hemoglobin so that it can be expelled. Until the immature liver can do this fast enough, yellow pigment, or bilirubin, builds up in the tissues. When the bilirubin level gets very high, brain damage can result. So jaundiced babies are watched carefully.

The chances of jaundice are increased when the mother has received certain drugs – including aspirin, tranquilizers, diuretics, antibiotics, steroids, and sulpha drugs – when labor has been induced or accelerated with an oxytocin intravenous drip, and when she has had epidural anesthesia.

Treatment of jaundice

The treatment for jaundice is abundant fluids, which means breastfeeding ad lib. Phototherapy can also be used, which entails putting the baby under bright artificial light to reduce serum bilirubin in the blood and tissues. Bilirubin is light-sensitive. An ordinary fluorescent lamp is usually placed over the baby, who is blindfolded so that the eyes cannot be damaged. If you are at home, you can achieve the same effect by lying your baby naked in warm sunlight in the garden or on the terrace. Research on the value of light treatment was started after a nurse noticed that babies put by a window, where sunlight streamed in on them, had less jaundice than others who were in cribs away from the light.

It has been observed that delayed passage of meconium, the first contents of the baby's bowels, is associated with higher levels of bilirubin. Meconium is passed sooner when a baby is breastfed frequently from birth. So the best way of preventing jaundice is to start nursing shortly after birth and to nurse often without any supplementation.

It used to be assumed that jaundiced babies should be given water, but research has demonstrated that there is no benefit in this for breastfed babies. Though supplementary water does not prevent jaundice, mothers are often told that they should persuade their babies to take water "just in case". But giving anything at all in addition to your own milk interferes with the smooth start of breastfeeding, and may reduce milk production and get the baby hooked on the bottle. On the other hand, a jaundiced baby is usually sleepy and may need to be awakened for nursing every two hours during the day.

Breastmilk jaundice

There is a special, and rare, kind of jaundice called "breastmilk jaundice", where a mother's milk causes a rise in bilirubin in her baby's tissues. This is often over-diagnosed, but if the pediatrician thinks that your baby has this, and that your milk is responsible, there is still no need to give up breastfeeding entirely. You will need to interrupt breastfeeding for, at most, twenty-four hours, to enable the bilirubin level to go down; you may have to repeat this in successive weeks.

While the baby is being bottle-fed you should express your milk regularly in order to keep up your milk supply. It may be that the baby can be fed expressed breastmilk from a milk bank, instead of infant formula, while you are unable to nurse her.

Babies with Handicaps

For any baby who finds it difficult to get the neuromuscular coordination going that is needed for sucking and swallowing, learning to breastfeed is a challenge.

To be able to breastfeed, the mother has to establish a good milk supply with a lively milk ejection reflex. That means expressing milk regularly to make up for the baby's feeble sucking – either after each nursing or in place of nursing while the baby is being tube-fed or is fed by bottle or spoon. It is possible to lactate for months on end using expression alone, though it is tedious and you have to be very committed to do it.

The baby cannot shape a bottle nipple in the same way she can breast tissue, which is beautifully flexible. If a baby has difficulty in coordinating tongue, jaw, swallowing, and breathing movements, it may be easier to breastfeed, because she can mold the breast into the most convenient shape.

Down syndrome and cerebral palsy

A baby with Down syndrome or cerebral palsy, for whom neuromuscular control is hard, breastfeeding may be best if you can get over the initial difficulties.

Some Down syndrome babies breastfeed well from the start. Others take a while to get coordinated. Some never manage it at all, usually because they do not suck easily – they are often the ones who have a heart problem as well, as 50 per cent of these babies do.

In the first two weeks, concentrate on initiating lactation by expression. Then you will have time on hand for helping the baby to get used to breastfeeding.

Cleft palate

A baby with a cleft palate often cannot easily form a nipple shape with the breast because she cannot create a vacuum between the breast and her mouth. If the cleft is not central, or if it is short, she can block the cleft with the breast. Even so, you may need to start breastfeeding wearing a flexible nipple

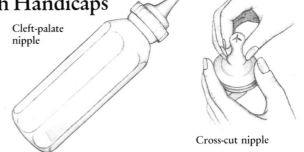

Cleft-palate nipple

Cross-cut nipple

Some babies with cleft palates *can suck from an elongated nipple. There are also special cross-cut nipples or you can cross-cut a regular nipple.*

shield. It helps sometimes if the baby is fitted with a small plastic plate to correct the shape of the hard palate. But babies usually need the sensation of the breast against the palate and become distressed if they do not have this.

If you can maintain your milk supply until after the baby has had the operation to repair the palate, you may be able to start breast-feeding afterward. Immediately following the operation, before you begin nursing, you can give your baby expressed milk using a bottle with an elongated nipple or a nipple which has been cross-cut. There are many different kinds of nipple on the market. The Cleft Palate Foundation can let you have information about these and will give advice about nursing (see page 156).

When you nurse your baby you may be anxious that your milk comes down her nose before she swallows. This does not matter. If she coughs or chokes, nurse more slowly.

Cardiac defect

A baby who has a heart defect and metabolic illness may be able to breastfeed. One who is receiving oxygen therapy can breastfeed with a nasal catheter still in place. But the neonatologist and cardiologist may advise you to bottle-feed, believing that breastfeeding is more stressful for the baby. Research has shown, however, that for pre-term babies breastfeeding does not use up more energy, providing that the milk is flowing well.

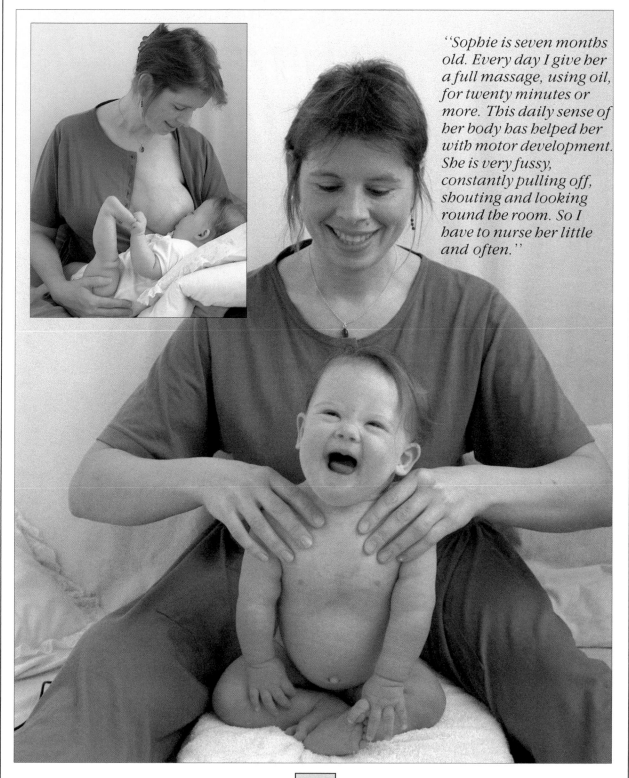

"Sophie is seven months old. Every day I give her a full massage, using oil, for twenty minutes or more. This daily sense of her body has helped her with motor development. She is very fussy, constantly pulling off, shouting and looking round the room. So I have to nurse her little and often."

The Baby's Emotional Experience

MOST OF A BABY'S LIFE has to do with nursing and all the things connected with nursing. There is hunger and the longing for food, the excitement of taking the breast into the mouth, pleasure as milk squirts against the soft palate, the satisfaction of sucking and swallowing, and the delicious feeling as the milk goes down and the baby's tummy becomes full. Then there are all the processes involved in digestion: sensations of pressure, bubbles of gas, rhythms of the tightening of the gut, and the surprising events that occur at the other end, producing warm liquid and solid matter as if by magic.

The pleasure of nursing

When you watch a baby at the breast who is enjoying a feeding, it is clear that all her attention, every muscle and nerve fiber, every atom of her being, is focused on a thrilling and sensuous activity. Dr. Donald Winnicott, a pediatrician and psychiatrist, once remarked that when nursing is going well, "the whole of the emerging personality is engaged." Yet nursing can be done mechanically, just like filling up the tank with gasoline. If, for example, a mother is not paying her baby any attention and is thinking of other things, then it may be so boring for the baby that it is a relief for her to cry with anger and frustration.

Communication of feelings

Bottle-feeding can be a fulfilling experience for a baby, too, when it is done with sensitivity and closeness. An important element is the mother's attention, and the way in which she concentrates it on her baby, at least intermittently, as they look into each other's eyes. With breastfeeding, however, an additional part of the overall experience is the taste, smell, and feel of the breast from which the delicious milk flows freely.

Everything a mother is feeling as the baby sucks at her breast is part of the baby's experience as well. These feelings are communicated spontaneously through her eyes and mouth, in the way she holds her baby, by the movements of her body and in her voice and her breathing. From all that a mother gives her baby in these ways, the baby begins to learn about life and to have rich and varied emotional experiences.

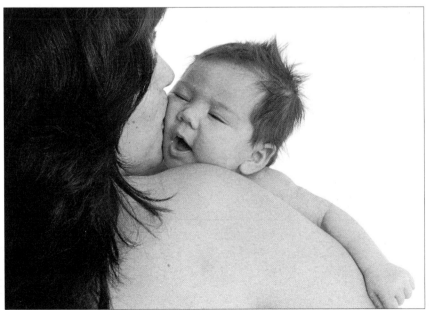

When a baby is at the breast (right) *he is unaware of anything that is going on around him as, with eyes tightly closed, he is enveloped by a sensuous activity that is totally satisfying – the bliss of suckling.*

A baby enjoys being showered with kisses *and having a big bear-hug (left). Knowing that she is loved is an important part of a baby's emotional experience and makes her feel secure and happy.*

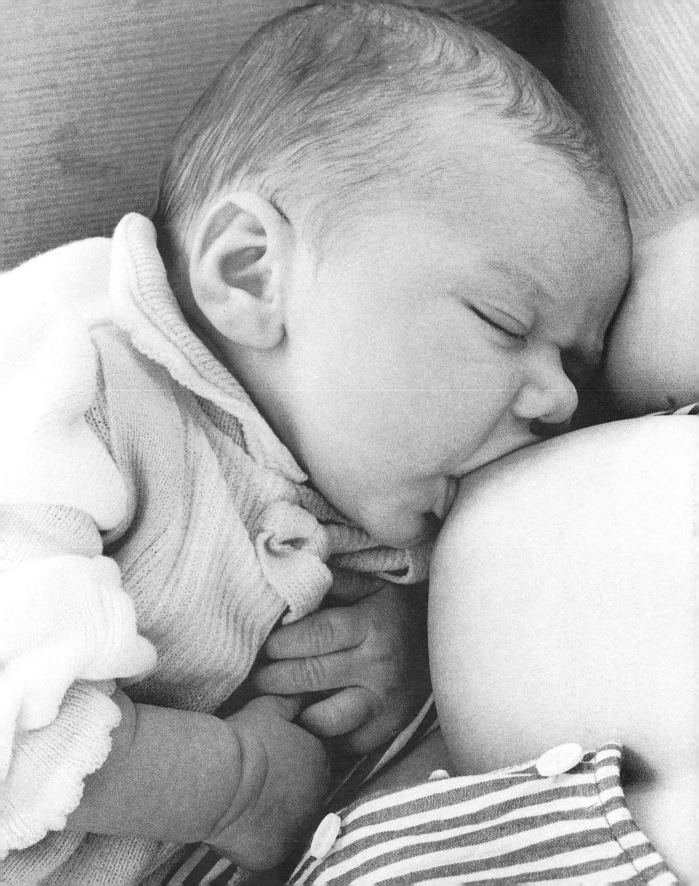

Managing Your Time

When you first have a baby you may feel that you will never have time to fit into your waking hours everything you need to do. A new baby can be a full-time job – and more, since there is no point at which you can leave. You are on duty twentyfour hours of the day, and the difference between day and night becomes blurred. You may feel you have to rush feedings or put off the baby with a skimped feeding because you must do something else, such as cooking a meal, but you will soon discover that the baby always seems to be aware of this and gets cross.

It is impossible to force schedules on a small baby. And even though you can discover the baby's rhythms, this is very difficult in the first three months. Babies often sleep and wake at unexpected times and need your immediate attention as their mouths open and, with eyes still tightly closed, they grope for the breast, knowing only that they want to be nursed, and quickly.

Feeling guilty

Some women feel almost guilty about sitting down and nursing a baby because they ought to be cooking a meal, washing the dishes, doing the laundry, making the beds, tidying the living room, or vacuuming the floor. It is as if what they are doing is self-indulgent, or of secondary importance to housework. Other people, including an otherwise loving partner, may expect life to go on more or less as before the baby came, since in all cultures it is usually assumed that women have a natural ability for housework and can cope in all situations.

Getting extra help

However much help you had before, you need more now. When you are breastfeeding you are not resting – even if you are lying down or curled up on a sofa. If you have never had much help from your partner there will have to be a massive change in the way you share the work between you. He will

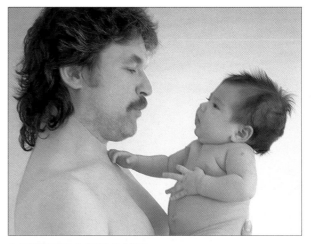

A FATHER & HIS BABY

1 *A man spends time with his baby to get to know her when he could be doing other things.*

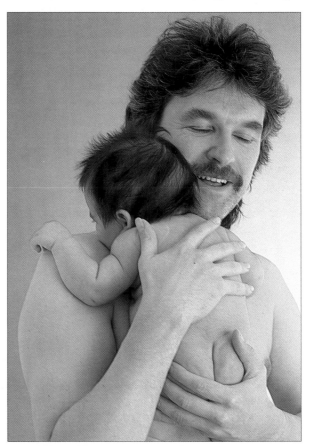

2 *In caring for his baby, he may discover a deeper tenderness in himself.*

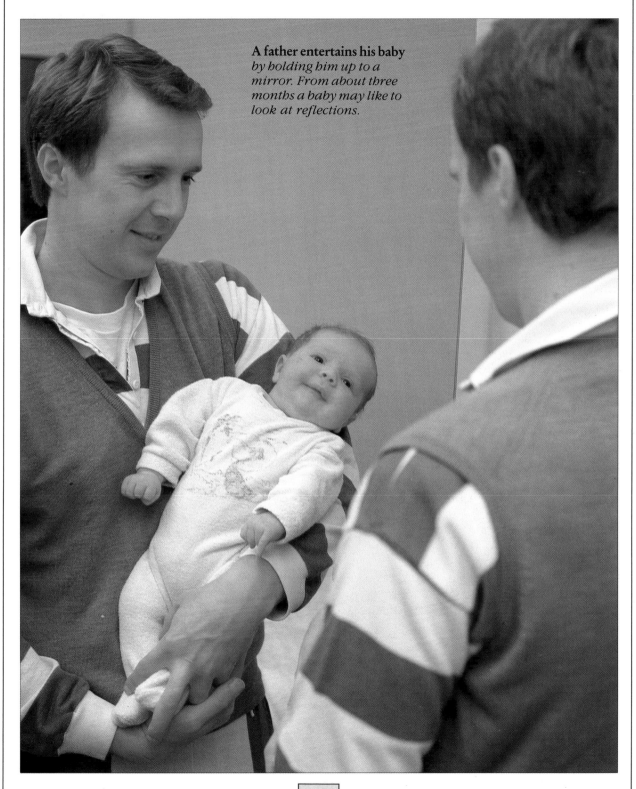

A father entertains his baby *by holding him up to a mirror. From about three months a baby may like to look at reflections.*

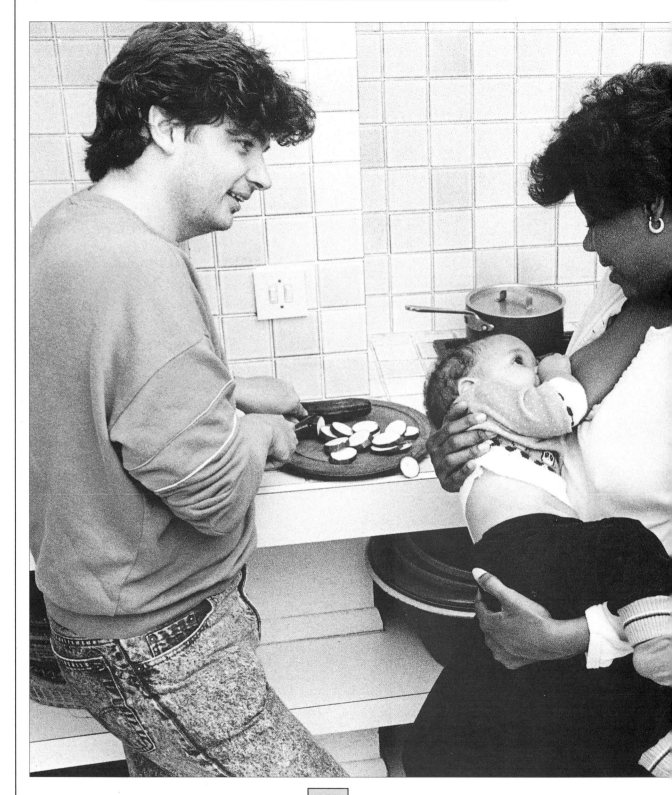

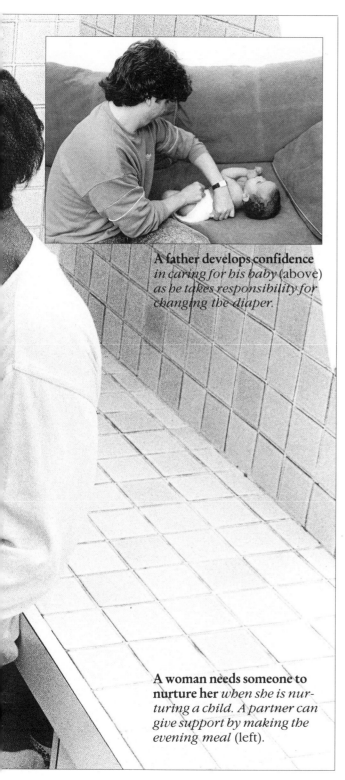

A father develops confidence *in caring for his baby* (above) *as he takes responsibility for changing the diaper.*

A woman needs someone to nurture her *when she is nurturing a child. A partner can give support by making the evening meal* (left).

have to take over jobs he is not accustomed to doing – and things that he may protest he has never learned to do or does not do at all well.

A father's role

Breastfeeding in no way makes a father superfluous. A woman who is nurturing a baby needs to be nurtured herself, and her partner may be the person who can do this best. There are many other things a baby needs beside feeding – to be held up to smile at the baby in the mirror; to be changed, bathed, and comforted, to be bounced, patted, rocked and talked to – and there are many extra jobs because of the baby's presence. Shared parenting means that a father takes on all these tasks. It is hard work but it can be for him an enriching experience.

When friends and relatives visit, enlist their help, too. Let them admire the baby, then ask them to do something to help while you nurse. You do not have to entertain them as before.

Time for playing

If you do not have any help, you will find that you have little time for talking to, singing, or playing with your baby, and providing stimulating things for her to explore with her senses. When you do these things you introduce a child to life with its richly varied experiences. You help a baby to develop into a human being. A woman alone has little time to spare for this, just as a woman with older children at home may have her whole day taken up with simply caring for them and cleaning and tidying up after them.

Other cultures organize childcare better. There are co-mothers to share childcare and members of the extended family to take over responsibility. In an industrialized society mothers must often bear total responsibility for the children, socially isolated in what is virtually solitary confinement. Meanwhile fathers often miss out on the early weeks and months of their children's development, not just because they are away from home, but because mothers are expected to know instinctively what to do with babies.

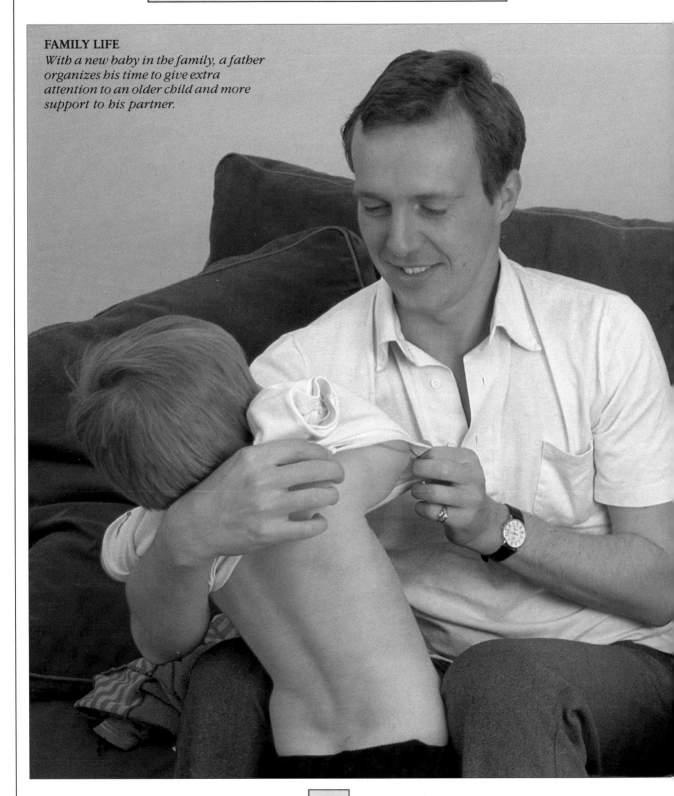

FAMILY LIFE
With a new baby in the family, a father organizes his time to give extra attention to an older child and more support to his partner.

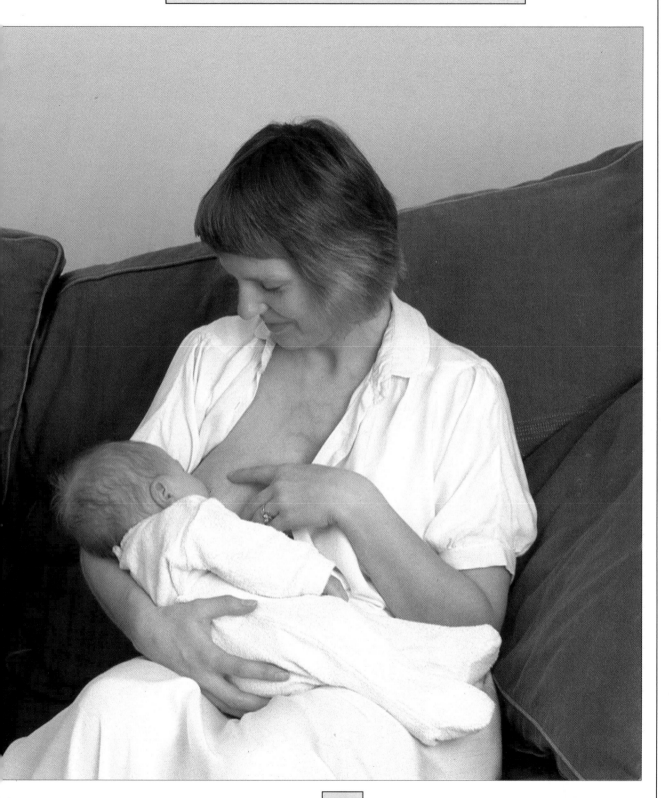

Your Needs

While keeping tuned to the baby's needs, it is important that you are also aware of your own needs. Most of the time the needs of a mother and her nursing baby overlap. The baby comes to the breast and the mother feels the warmth and prickling rush of the milk ejection reflex, and has satisfaction in holding the baby and knowing that he is receiving milk. Yet sometimes a mother needs space to be herself, apart from the baby.

Confidence in yourself

A woman who is breastfeeding needs, above all, confidence in herself. She needs to feel in control. It helps to have support from other people around you – your family and friends – people who also believe that you can nurture your child, and do not criticize you or undermine your faith in yourself. Those who give support should not try to take over the baby and replace you, or in any way compete for the baby's love. They are there ready to help when you need it, but respect the bond that links a mother and her baby, and realize that you will grow to understand each other.

A little advice goes a very long way. In fact, advice is often wrong. And even if the facts are right, advice can be destructive, and your attempts to follow it distort the subtle relationship you have with your baby. New mothers are often bombarded with advice, especially from their own mothers, who intervene with advice about how they could organize their lives better with the new baby. They worry that the baby is too demanding; they worry when he cries, and want to say or do something that will help. They may say and do the wrong things and leave you feeling a failure. But if you follow your own instincts, you will be doing what is right for your baby and your self confidence will grow.

Time for yourself

A woman may need some regular time – however short – away from the baby. Much depends on the birth experience. If this was

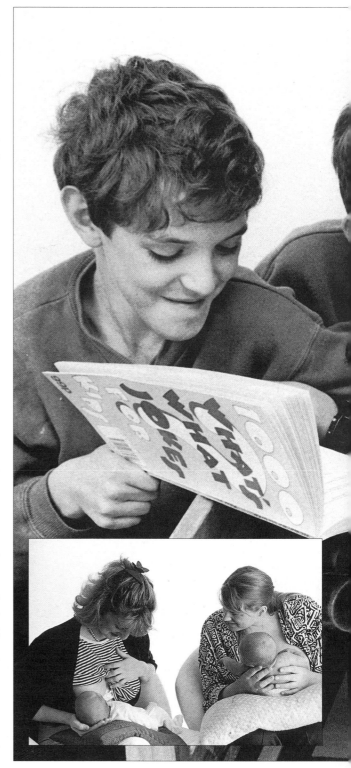

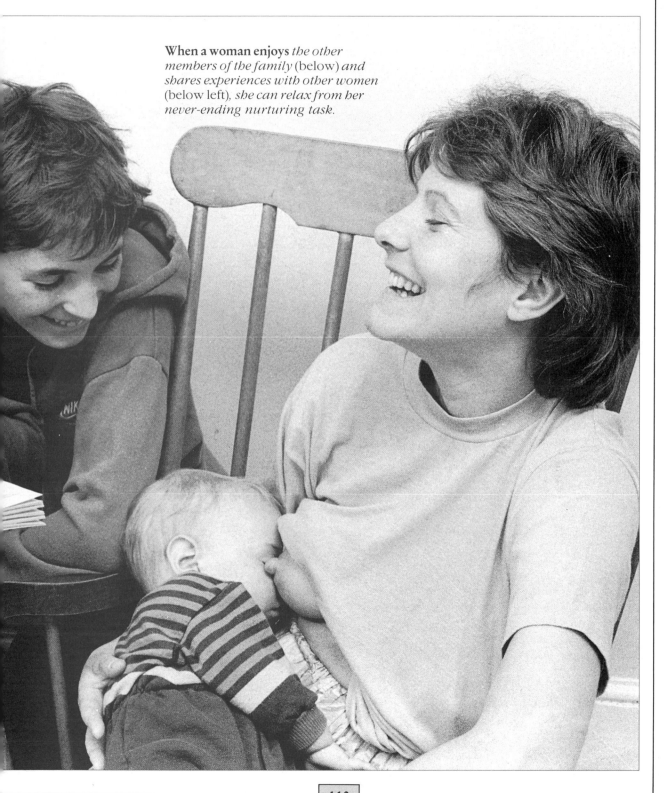

When a woman enjoys *the other members of the family* (below) *and shares experiences with other women* (below left), *she can relax from her never-ending nurturing task.*

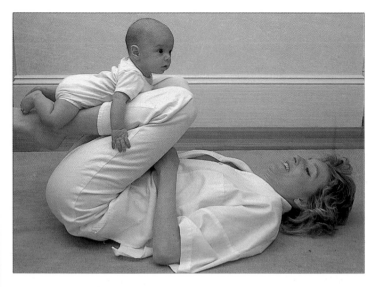

Exercises to tone your muscles *can be done so that the baby enjoys them, too* (left). *With the small of your back pressed flat against the floor, swing the baby on your legs to strengthen your tummy muscles.*

good, and she emerged feeling strong and in control, she can relate to the baby and get "in tune" from the very beginning.

If, on the other hand, she feels in any way disempowered by what she has been through, she needs both uninterrupted time alone with her baby, and space to be by herself without any demands being made of her. The timing of this is a matter for sensitive adjustment in the pattern of baby care through the twenty-four hours. It is vital for her to take space for herself wherever she can find it, rather than wearing herself out in struggling to be a "good" mother. If she is to do this, she needs another adult able and willing to take over everyday chores for her.

Change of environment

Any woman with a baby or toddler benefits from a regular change in her environment, too. In one sense, a breastfeeding mother is in bondage to her baby, linked in mind and body and through her endocrine system and all the complex emotions she has about her baby. Much of this bondage is pleasurable, but with all of us there come times when we need to escape from the intensity and the demanding nature of this experience, and talk to adults, for example, or do something entirely different.

Many women are deprived of this opportunity, especially in the first year of a child's life, because our society is not organized for mothers and babies. Thousands of women with children are also caught in a poverty trap and have to use all their resources just to keep going from day to day.

If this is how it is for you, and there is a chance to get out of the house regularly, take it. When you can get into the fresh air and have a change of scene, do not hesitate. Many women say that even a walk to the store, in spite of bad weather, or just chatting with other mothers while waiting at the school gate, brings relief from the unremitting hard work of caring for a baby.

In good weather have a stroll in the park, arrange a picnic with other mothers and children in the garden, or a trip together into the countryside or to the beach. You have the advantage as a breastfeeding mother of being able to nurse your baby wherever you are. All you have to do is to find somewhere to sit, open up, and let him latch on while you relax and enjoy the change of scene. When women share with each other and do things together you realize that you are not alone, that other women feel as you do, and that by joining together you are stronger and have more confidence in yourself.

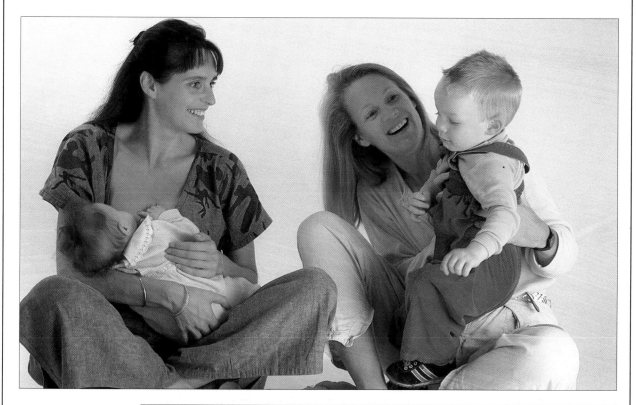

A woman can best cope with the challenges *of motherhood when she is part of a network of women with children* (above and right), *who are honest and open about their negative as well as their positive feelings, and who give each other emotional support and reassurance.*

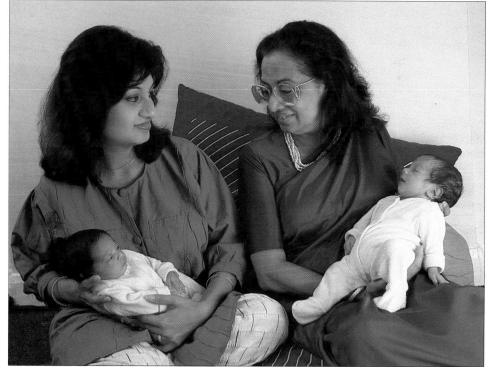

Fitting in with the Family

When your baby is born your older child may feel replaced and rejected. She needs to know that you still love her and that you are not cutting short your time with her because of the new baby.

You can prepare your other children by discussing the birth and breastfeeding well before the baby comes, and by showing them pictures of babies being born and at their mother's breast. If you have to change sleeping arrangements or routines, or want older children to be toilet-trained or to start playgroup, nursery, or school, do this several months before the baby comes, or leave it until six months or so after the birth to allow your child to settle down again.

Sibling rivalry

When you are breastfeeding you may find that an older child wants to suck, too, and to be held and cuddled. Sometimes children pretend they are babies again for a while. Responding positively to your children's need of you, assuring them of your love, and going along with this as if it was a pleasant game, is more likely to help them feel secure than if you push them to "act their age."

An older child may prove very demanding when you have a baby at the breast, asking for a drink of water, doing things that are dangerous or very noisy, or even throwing a tantrum. You can make sure that the room is completely safe and prepare a favourite drink or snack in readiness.

Once you are sure you have the baby well latched on you can cuddle an older child, tell a story, or sing together, so that breastfeeding gives you all a special closeness. If you usually nurse in one room, keep a store of playthings there reserved for these special times. The older child will know that when the baby is at the breast it is a sign to open that particular toy cupboard.

Sibling rivalry is normal. But there are many ways in which you can help your child to grow through this phase.

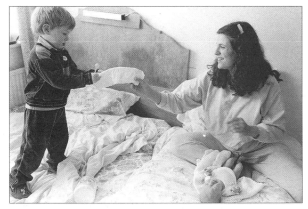

A HELPFUL TODDLER

1 *A small child helps by getting things for the baby. She lets him know she appreciates this.*

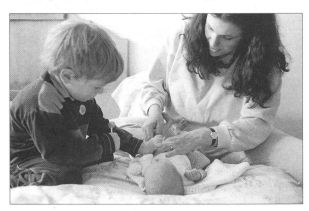

2 *He holds a diaper in place around the wriggling baby. By collaborating in this task, he learns a caring gentleness.*

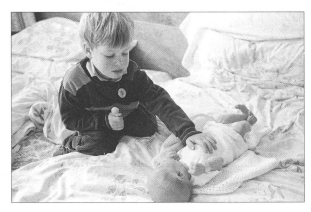

3 *Given the responsibility of looking after the baby, he pats her gently and is delighted when she gazes up at him.*

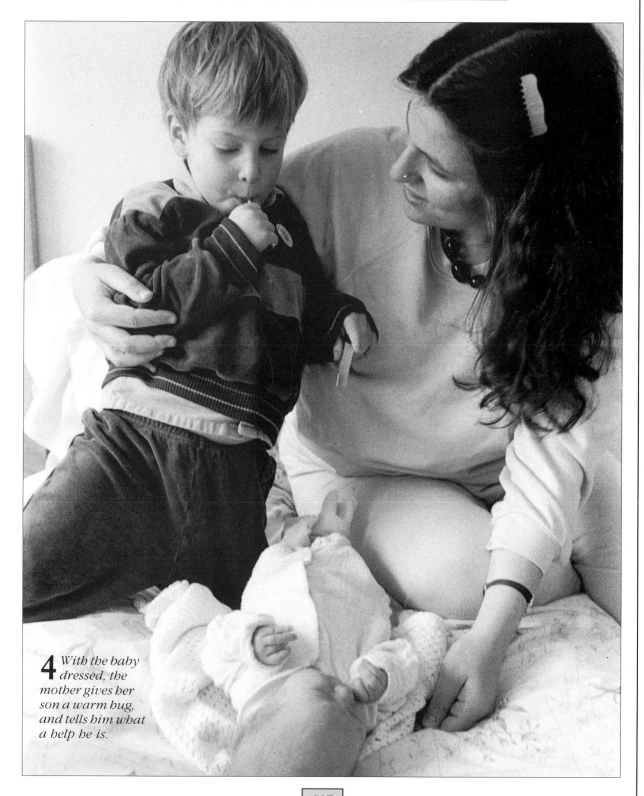

4 *With the baby dressed, the mother gives her son a warm hug, and tells him what a help he is.*

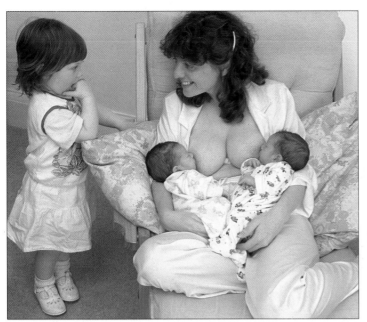

THE NEEDS OF AN OLDER CHILD

1 *When you are concentrating on caring for the new baby, your other child may feel very left out. Be sensitive to her feelings. There is no room in your arms for her and she is bereft – especially when there are twins!*

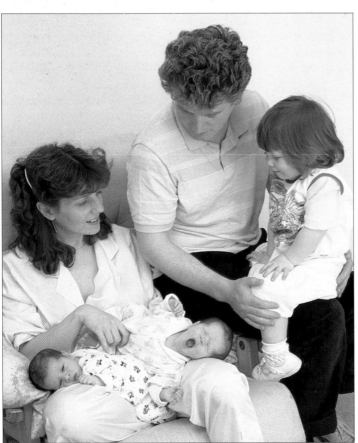

2 *When there is another adult you can trust, who gives extra love and attention to the older child, this helps her feel more secure. Instead of feeling that she has been usurped, she begins to enjoy the new additions to the family.*

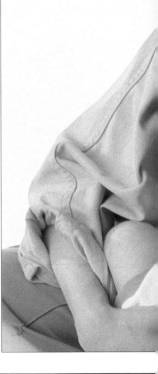

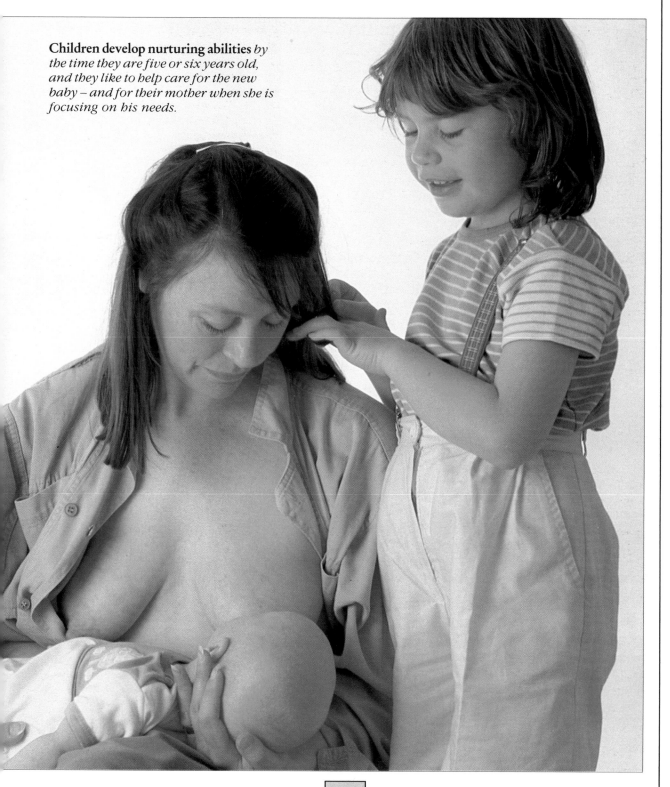

Children develop nurturing abilities *by the time they are five or six years old, and they like to help care for the new baby – and for their mother when she is focusing on his needs.*

"I should have stuck to goldfish."

When a baby cries and fusses and demands all of your time, attention, and energy, you may feel like dumping her in the wastepaper basket. You are not the only mother who feels like this. Others do too – even apparently calm, happy, competent mothers. If you have had nothing to do with babies before and your only experience of caring for anything was your pet kitten or puppy, or even less demanding creatures like goldfish, there will probably be times when you wish you had never taken on responsibility for this unreasonable, demanding, noisy, angry little baby.

The fretting time

The evening is when it all starts for many babies. They become restless and cross, and nothing keeps them happy for more than a few minutes at a time. One mother calls the period from 6 to 7pm "the arsenic hour." She is lucky – some babies go on fussing much longer than that. By that time of day you are ready to slow down and have a rest. You look forward to a quiet meal with your partner. But it is not to be.

Most babies who are past the immediate newborn stage and are not yet three or four months old have an irritable spell at some time in the day, when they want frequent nursing and like to return to the first breast after they have had a long session at both sides already. You then put them down to sleep and they are awake again, ready to nurse, within half an hour.

You may wonder whether you have enough milk to satisfy your baby. However, this fretting time is nothing to do with either the quantity or the quality of your milk. It is rather that the baby is supercharged and in a state of nervous excitability in which she needs to discharge tension by twitching, crying, jerking, wriggling, squirming, and sucking.

Offering distractions

Any and everything you do to try and help your baby may seem wrong. Some things work for a short while: more interesting surroundings, something that catches her attention, such as looking at herself in a mirror, gazing at a ticking clock, or watching older children playing. Soothing music sometimes helps, but the baby may be crying so loudly that she cannot hear it. Carrying her around in a sling may be effective for longer still, especially if you keep moving. You may also

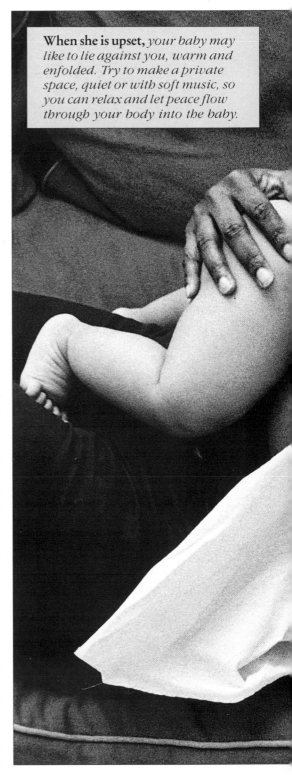

When she is upset, *your baby may like to lie against you, warm and enfolded. Try to make a private space, quiet or with soft music, so you can relax and let peace flow through your body into the baby.*

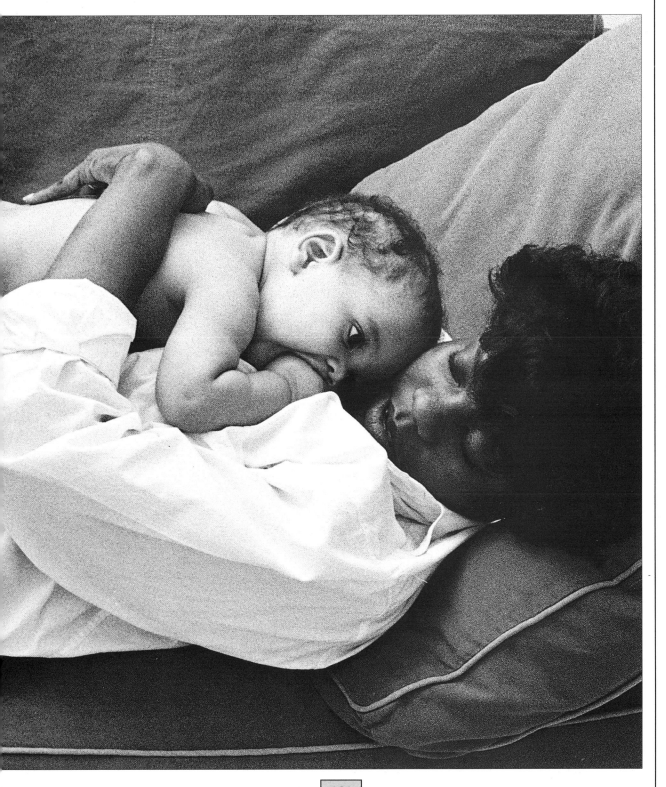

find that lying down in a darkened room with the baby lying spreadeagled on your body, where she can hear the beating of your heart and feel the comforting warmth of your flesh, helps. Or you could try simply rocking your baby and gently patting her back.

Placing a baby in a warm bath is a good way of helping her to relax, so it is sensible to plan bath-time for that time of the day or evening in which you know your baby is most likely to be in this restless state. Another effective way of soothing a baby whose desperate crying is already reduced to sobs, is to rest your head against hers and to hum or intone so that the baby not only hears the sound of your voice, but the resonance. A deep, low tone is often best, but you can vary it. As the baby relaxes, the reverberating hum can turn into singing. Finding a way to soothe your baby is a matter of trial and error, always letting her lead the way, and it can take weeks to discover what works best.

Determined to cry

But then, just when you think that you have found an answer to her distress, you do something else that starts her crying again. You move and she is startled. You speak and she grimaces. You change position to try to get her more comfortable and she flinches and then yells even louder. It may seem impossible to know what to do to help your baby. She won't settle with you and yet if you leave her alone she cries as if totally abandoned, and that is agony for you, too.

Someone may tell you to put her in her crib and let her cry herself to sleep. But if you put a frantically screaming baby in her crib, she is likely to cry more. She will fall asleep eventually, when exhausted, but she really needs to be calm before she can sleep peacefully.

The baby sleeps

At last the baby falls asleep and you breathe a sigh of relief. All is quiet for fifteen or twenty minutes – an hour if you are fortunate. And then the baby makes a convulsive movement and starts to cry irritably again. If you respond quickly, patting her bottom as she lies in her crib, and just offering a reassuring presence, she may drift off to sleep again. Or it may be obvious that she is too upset for this and wants the comfort of the breast again. When you pick her up before she is in a full spate of crying, soothing her by wrapping her in a blanket or big towel, and offer the breast, she may at last suck rhythmically, relax, and drop off to sleep.

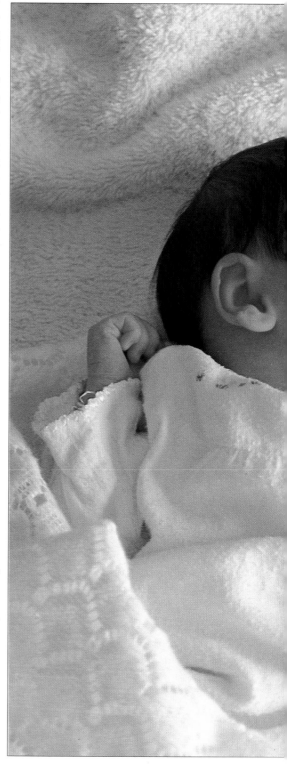

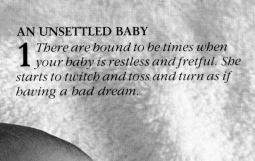

AN UNSETTLED BABY

1 *There are bound to be times when your baby is restless and fretful. She starts to twitch and toss and turn as if having a bad dream.*

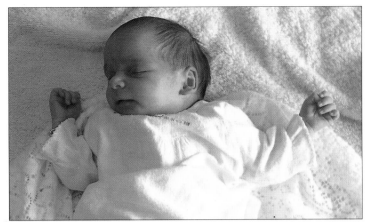

2 *She makes little jerky movements and wriggles, unable to settle. You watch her anxiously.*

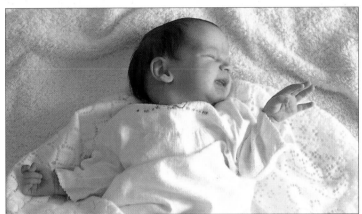

3 *Perhaps if you ignore her she will settle. Other people tell you to put her in another room.*

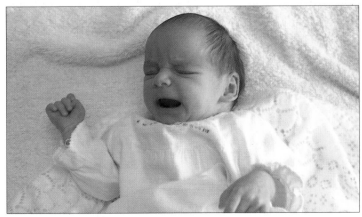

4 *But you can't bear knowing that she is uncomfortable. She starts to cry. You pick her up.*

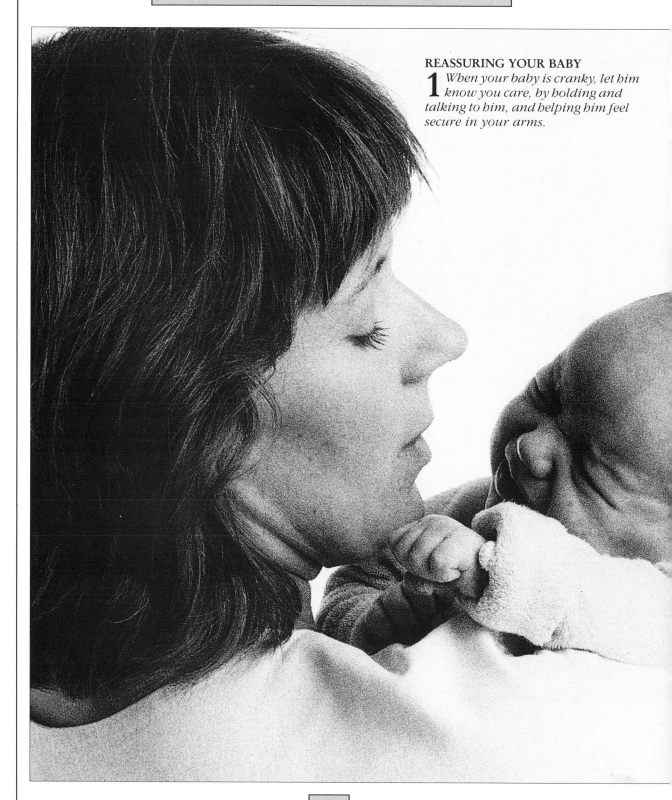

REASSURING YOUR BABY

1 *When your baby is cranky, let him know you care, by holding and talking to him, and helping him feel secure in your arms.*

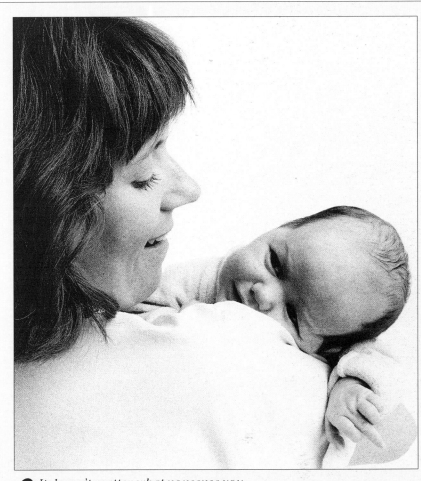

2 *It doesn't matter what nonsense you say, or what silly sounds you make. The baby will know you are telling him that you love him.*

CALMING A CRYING BABY

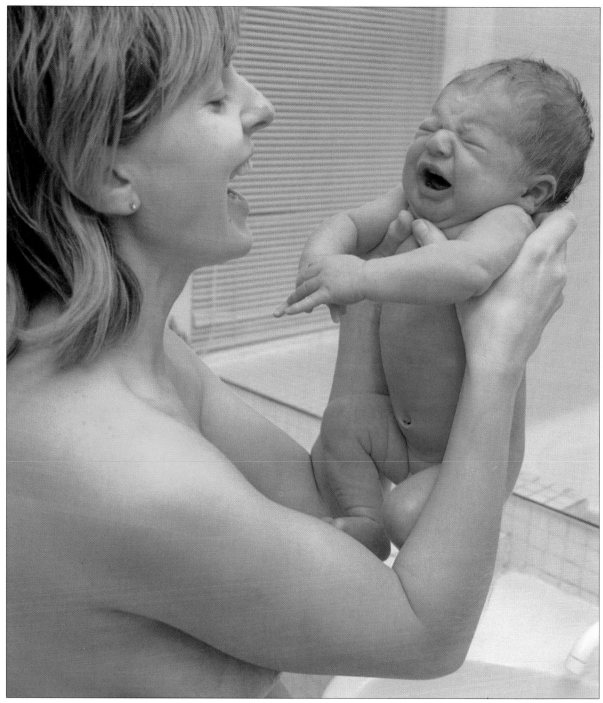

1 *When your baby cries, try not to let your feelings of anger and despair take over. Keep calm and reassure him by talking or singing.*

This is the time when, no longer having to provide a split-second response to your baby's need of you, you can reclaim a little space and relax in the knowledge that, in spite of your doubts, you are a good enough mother, and can enjoy a new freedom.

At three months

By the time your baby is ten to twelve weeks old, she will already have definite ways of letting you know what she wants. If you put her to the breast and she does not wish to nurse, she may go rigid, arch her back, throw up her arms, and protest loudly. Or she may take the opportunity to play with your breasts if she is in the mood. Breasts are splendid play-things because they are soft and bouncy. She may lick the nipple or tickle it with her lips, try to chew it, or even grab and bite you – all the time watching you. She finds your reactions very interesting. When she is rough with you, withdraw and tell her quite firmly that she must not do it again as you do not like it. She will soon understand.

Wake and sleep states

When your baby wakes, but is still sodden with sleep, she may shift into a more comfortable position, or if on her front, stick her bottom in the air, and creep forward with a kind of caterpillar propulsion until she has her head resting against something firm – the top of the crib or a wall or cupboard – and then close her eyes again and have another snooze. If you pick her up before she has had this extra sleep she may be irritable.

A baby who has had a good sleep may wake refreshed and want simply to be assured of your presence. Then she starts to explore the surroundings and to play. She waves her fist in the air and watches it with cross-eyed concentration. She brings her hands together, and each gropes for the other, but often misses. She kicks, finds a foot with her hand, holds it for an exciting moment, and then loses it again. If a mirror is set alongside her, she will turn and watch the other baby with great seriousness. Then she chuckles.

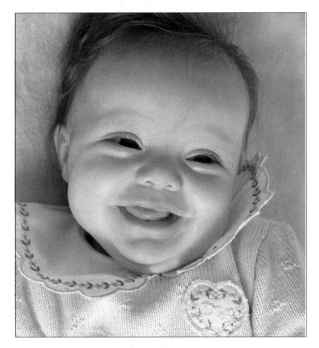

Some babies are sociable *(above)*, *while others are more thoughtful and contemplative* (below). *As they develop, outgoing babies become quiet if they have interesting things to explore. Placid babies become sociable when with a trusted person.*

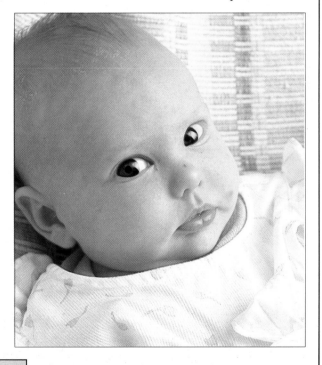

When in an exuberant mood the baby talks to anyone and anything around – a picture on the wall, a chair, and herself – with little whoops and chortles of delight. If she gets bored, this conversation becomes querulous and there is a note of impending trouble. When you are busy with something else and half listening to her, you know immediately that she is ready for a different occupation.

A baby likes anything hanging on a string or ribbon – a mobile, a jingling necklace, or a bell – that can be swiped at with hands or feet. You can make a simple mobile by threading foil cupcake cups with thread and suspending them from a wire coathanger over the back of a chair. Your baby will try to get everything into her mouth to explore it fully, so it is vital that there is nothing on which she can choke or which can scratch or bruise her.

Understanding your baby

There are times when the baby seems to be furious with you for no reason. She cries at the top of her voice and whatever you do is wrong. Other people ask: "Is she hungry?...too hot?...too cold?...Have you changed her diaper?" And then suddenly, as you cuddle her close, her anger vanishes.

But after a while she starts to cry again. You know your baby well enough by now to realize that these are signs that she is over-tired and that even if you are not successful at comforting her, the message that you are *trying* to give comfort is important. Eventually the cries become sobs and you are able to soothe her to sleep.

A baby may also be restless because she is about to empty her bowels and is concentrating on something inside her which disturbs her. Then, with an expression of intense satisfaction, she holds her breath, grunts, and you hear the unmistakable sounds of a stool being passed.

Over the last weeks you have watched your baby carefully and you know, as no one else quite understands, all these very different emotional and physical states. You understand your baby.

RHYTHMS OF A BABY

1 By four months your baby is happy to lie and play by herself for a while when she wakes (right). She may take great delight in discovering her own foot, and be in no hurry to nurse. You hear gurgles, coos, and squeals as she experiments with different sounds.

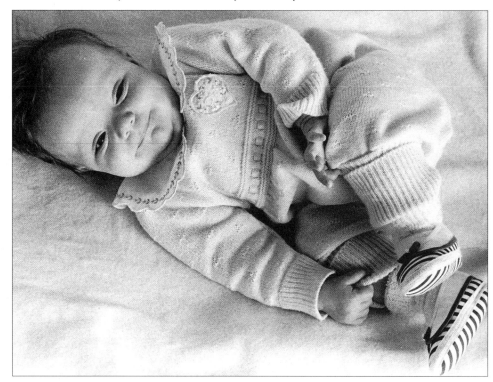

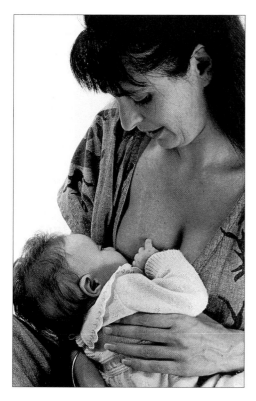

2 *When she is ready to nurse, she lets you know with an urgent cry. She knows exactly how to latch on and sucks with relish (left). Her excitement at the start gives way to blissful relaxation.*

3 *After being awake for a few hours, she becomes tearful (right). You know she is overtired and needs to be soothed so that she can go to sleep. But she finds it difficult to relax and is not easily comforted.*

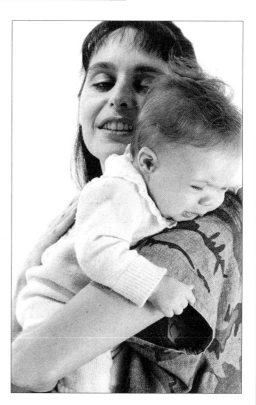

4 *Eventually you are able to soothe her off to sleep (right). She sleeps soundly, even though there may be noise all around her. And when she wakes afresh, she will be bursting with renewed energy.*

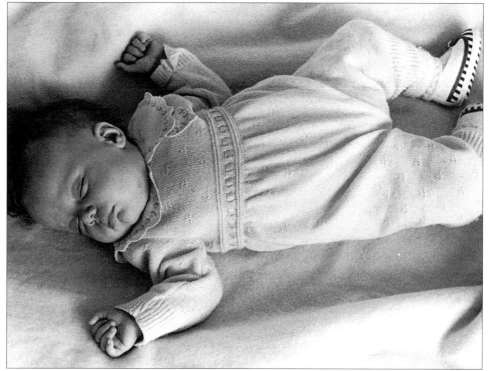

The Older Baby

As YOUR BABY DEVELOPS, nursing becomes fun for you both. It is like a lively conversation with lots of eye contact, smiles, giggles, and gurgles. Your baby may murmur and talk to you, too, imitating the cadences of your own speech, stopping so that you can have a turn, and then replying.

The experienced nurser

An older baby knows exactly where the breast is and homes in on it through layers of clothing with unerring aim. He may indicate in a peremptory manner that you should lift your sweater or undo your shirt, and then discover that he can do this himself and become adept at shifting clothing, and later still at undoing buttons, snaps, and zippers. This is the stage at which you may find your breasts suddenly bared in public!

Some babies experiment with acrobatic nursing. They like exploring the effect of different positions. Once fully mobile, a baby may latch on to a handy breast from any angle. He may crawl right up to you and nurse while still leaning against your body.

An older baby often comes into contact with other children. By continuing to breastfeed your baby, you are providing the immune properties of breastmilk, making him less likely to get colds, tummy upsets, and earaches. If your baby does catch a cold, however, it tends to be less severe than that of a baby fed with formula milk.

Teething

When the first tooth is about to come through, your baby's gum may be sore and he will like to gnaw and bite. He may want to suck at the breast more frequently for comfort, but if he tries to bite your nipple, take him off firmly and say "no". He will soon understand. Help your baby's teething with objects on which to bite: a teething ring, some zwieback or breadsticks, or a rattle of convenient size so that he can put a little of it in his mouth, and, if you are watching over him in case he chokes, easily grasped pieces of raw carrot or apple. Some teething rings can be filled with water and then frozen, which may feel good to your baby.

Attitudes of other people

You may find that other people disapprove of you breastfeeding your toddler. In Western society great emphasis is laid on babies progressing quickly to independence so that they can strike out in life and compete for success from an early age. People are often fearful that prolonged breastfeeding – into the second year of life and beyond – ties the baby to the mother so that this freedom never develops. In fact, the opposite is true. A child who is secure and confident of love, and who knows that the mother is ready to give immediate comfort, is better able to make explorations away from her. So if you are able to continue breastfeeding as long as your baby wants it, let him decide when to stop.

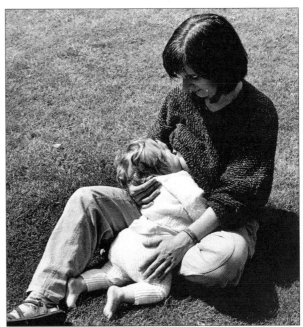

If you are sitting on the ground, *your toddler may make a beeline for your breast, and nurse leaning against you.*

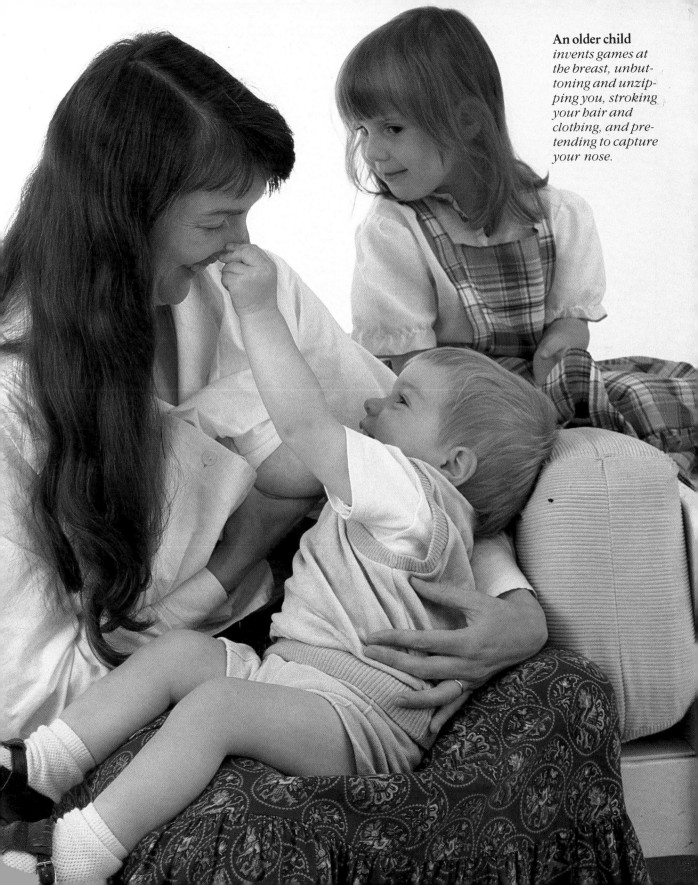

An older child *invents games at the breast, unbuttoning and unzipping you, stroking your hair and clothing, and pretending to capture your nose.*

Expressing Milk

It is useful to be able to express your breast-milk so that if you are away from your baby, someone else can give a bottle. If your breasts ever become engorged and uncomfortable, expressing milk will relieve them. There are several ways to express milk. Whichever method you use, have a clean towel handy to mop up any spills. If you intend to keep the milk, wash your hands first, and ensure that any equipment you use is sterilized.

To stimulate your milk ejection reflex, rest a hot towel or cloth against your breast. Then hold your breast underneath with one hand, and with the other hand, gently massage it, stroking from the outer edges of the breast in towards the nipple, all the way around as if following the spokes of a wheel. Or use a comb which you have drawn through soft soap – leave a cake of soap in a wet dish – rippling the comb from the outer margins of the breast in toward the areola.

Gravity flow

The simplest method of expressing milk is to lean forward so that your breasts hang down and then exert gentle pressure with your hands. This works well if you have a great deal of milk and a good milk ejection reflex. It may be the easiest way of releasing milk if your breasts feel very full, and if you just want to achieve a softer breast for the baby.

Hand expression

Hand expression is a simple technique when you know how. After massaging your breast, lean forward, supporting your breast underneath with the last three fingers of one hand and put the first finger of the other hand below the lower edge of the areola and your thumb above its upper edge. Relax your shoulder and neck muscles and breathe slowly. Then squeeze the breast rhythmically, as if you were squeezing toothpaste from a tube. To empty the breast thoroughly, move your fingers and thumb progressively around the outside of your breast, as if traveling

USING A NIPPLE SHIELD

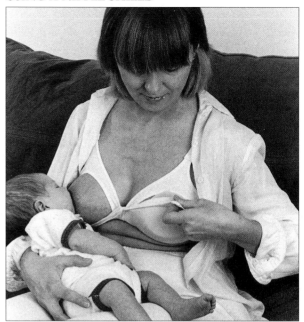

1 *To collect dripping milk while you nurse, put a nipple shield inside your nursing bra. Hook up the bra to keep the shield in place.*

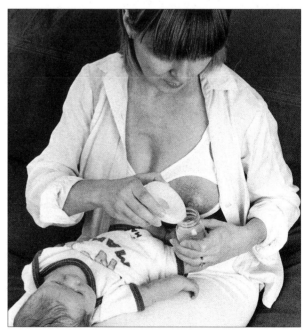

2 *When you can feel that it is almost full, remove it carefully and decant it into a jar for storage in a refrigerator or freezer.*

136

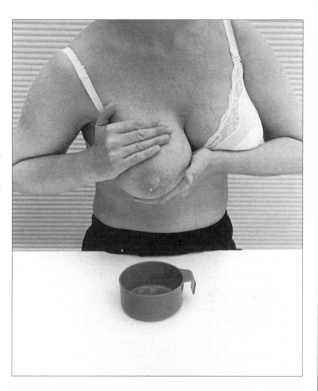

EXPRESSING MILK BY HAND

1 *To start the milk flow, support your breast with one hand and massage it with the other (right). Stroke down from your armpit toward the areola and then all around the globe of the breast.*

2 *Squeeze the lower part of the breast rhythmically with your thumb and index finger (below left), pressing deeply in on the glandular tissue to force the milk down.*

3 *Drops of milk glisten on the nipple and then milk spurts out in a steady stream (below right). Keep the flow going by gradually moving your hand around the outer edge of the areola.*

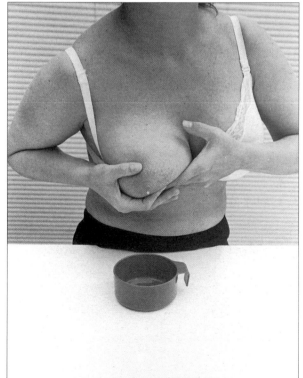

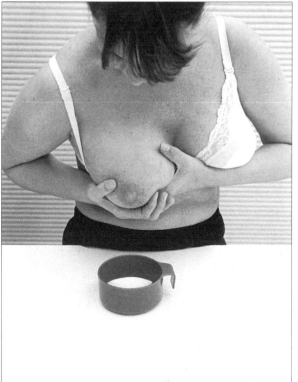

around the numbers on a clock face. Doing this frees the milk ducts so that you avoid a blockage of milk and inflammation.

Using a hand pump

The principle behind hand pumps is that of stimulating the hand action either with a piston movement from a cylinder or with a trigger action from a lever. Always moisten the breast before using the hand pump, to perfect the seal. The advantages of using hand pumps are that they can be quicker and easier than hand expression, and you may get more efficient milking of the breast.

Using an electric breast pump

An electric pump is more efficient still – almost as efficient as a baby. An electric pump needs to be started on its minimum suction setting, or the pull can be quite painful. As you get used to the sensation, gradually increase the suction. Treat your breasts gently, or you can cause nipple damage. Relax as you pump. Have a drink or a snack and read or

EXPRESSING & STORING MILK

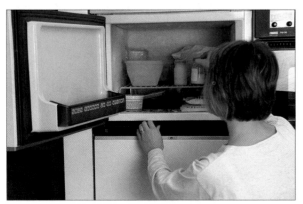

1 Wash your equipment in soapy water, rinse it well, and submerge it in a pan of water and boil the water for fifteen to twenty minutes to sterilize the equipment. Express your milk using the sterile pump.

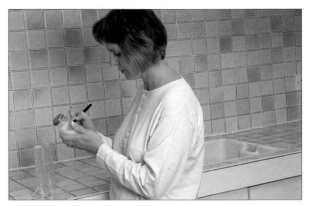

2 Pour the expressed breastmilk from the pump into a sterilized bottle, or a plastic bag which will fit inside a bottle. Seal it, and label it with the date and any other information you want to record for your future reference.

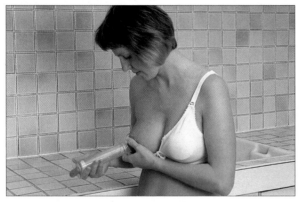

3 Place the milk in a freezer, where it will keep for up to six months. Or put it in a refrigerator – not the refrigerator door as the temperature there is warmer – for use within twentyfour hours.

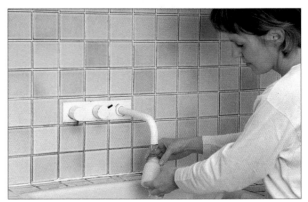

4 Thaw the frozen milk by holding it under a warm tap, then stand it in warm water. The milk will have separated but this does not matter. Use defrosted milk within a few hours.

listen to music. Reading this book, and looking at photographs of women breast-feeding, will help your milk ejection reflex.

If your baby is in special care you will need to use the pump every two to three hours at first. It helps to make a definite routine for this. Once you are at home, this will be difficult to do if you are under pressure to cook, clean, and run the house. So whenever possible arrange for other people to take this over.

Storing expressed milk

You can store breastmilk in the refrigerator for twentyfour hours – but not in the refrigerator door, as the temperature there is warmer – or in a freezer for up to six months. If you freeze milk, store it in plastic bottles on to which a rubber nipple can be screwed, or in plastic bags to fit in bottles. When defrosted it will have separated, but this does not matter – it is perfectly safe for the baby to drink. However, it should be used within a few hours. Never heat breastmilk as this destroys immune properties.

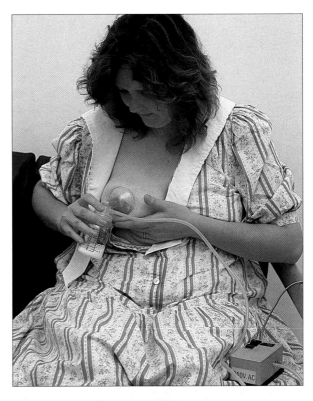

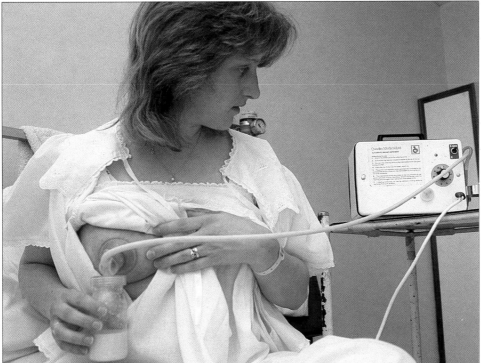

A small electric pump *is more effective than expressing by hand* (above). *You can control the strength of the suction with your finger.*

While in the hospital, *you can use a large electric pump* (left). *Breastfeeding groups and hospitals may supply one for home use.*

Sex & Breastfeeding

After you have had your baby you may be aching to get back to "normal" as soon as possible, or – on the other hand – you may enjoy the different way your body feels and looks. Breastfeeding obviously affects how you think about your body.

The pleasure of breastfeeding

Some women find that breastfeeding is, quite simply, a nurturing task, though a satisfying one, and gives a closeness to the baby which helps them to get to know him.

Other women discover – occasionally to their surprise – that breastfeeding is an elating experience. It brings to their bodies a pleasurable sensitivity, as well as a feeling of deep fulfillment. A woman who relishes breastfeeding may feel sexually aroused as her baby tugs and sucks. These feelings make some women feel ashamed and guilty. Yet it is normal to feel intense physical pleasure in breastfeeding, and sometimes even to have an orgasm as a result.

Most of us probably experience both these feelings at different times. We veer between simply managing to fit nursings into our busy lives, and experiencing them as deeply satisfying and even blissful.

Feelings about sex

In the early weeks – and sometimes months – of breastfeeding, many women are not sexually aroused in a way they have been previously, and do not enjoy genital sex. This is understandable. If you are facing difficulties in breastfeeding, for example, you probably do not feel at all good about your body and think of it as cumbersome and awkward. This in turn affects how you feel about sex. When you are trying to cope with breastfeeding problems you are likely to be anxious about them, and there is little or no time or energy for erotic sexual feelings.

For some women this reduction of libido persists right through the time they are lactating, probably as a result of the hormones

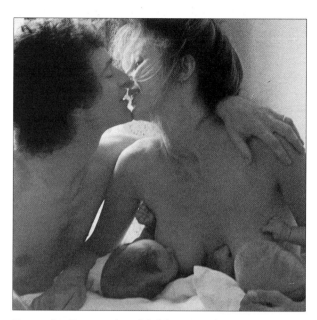

Breastfeeding can be a highly sensual experience, *not only for the mother, but shared with the father and babies too.*

that stimulate milk production. Your partner should be aware that when you know your baby is about to wake up to nurse, and you are listening for the first cry, or if you are worrying about the baby, you cannot concentrate on love-making. Without this mental focus any sexually arousing experience is just physical. Intense sexual excitement comes only when mind and body together have the same strong focus.

In the first weeks after childbirth you may be going through physical changes which cause pain or discomfort. An episiotomy, a cesarean incision, heavy blood loss, and physical exhaustion can all result in feeling that the last thing you want to think about at this time is sex.

However much you enjoy being a mother, your new role is bound to be stressful, too. There are all sorts of things to learn and challenges to confront. Your whole way of life changes. The relationship between you and your partner evolves, with your baby an important part of it. Worrying about not feeling sexually aroused makes this transition more difficult. Take one day at a time. If you had a good relationship before the baby came, you will find it again once you relax and the baby becomes part of the flow of your lives.

Effects of breastfeeding

While you are breastfeeding you may notice that your vagina is especially dry, even when you are sexually aroused. This is because during lactation the level of estrogen circulating in your body is lower than usual. If you wish to have intercourse, use a lubricant which either you or your partner can stroke into the dry tissues – you can make this a pleasurable part of love-making.

Pressure on your breasts may be painful while you are lactating, especially if they are full because a feeding is due shortly. Your partner should avoid putting weight on your breasts or squeezing them during love-making. The "missionary" position for intercourse may be uncomfortable for this reason.

Exploring new ways of love-making

You may often feel that you want to make love, but not to have intercourse. Love-making after childbirth enables you to explore together ways of arousing and satisfying each other which are far more complex and enriching than simple penetration and ejaculation. Some men who previously have ejaculated fast learn to prolong love-making so that it is much more satisfying for the woman, and in slowing down they become more gentle. A woman may discover she is capable of intense sexual arousal when all a partner is using is a little finger or a tenderly searching mouth.

A woman who is breastfeeding may feel that she doesn't want her partner making love to her breasts, even though she enjoyed it a great deal before the baby was born, and will again when lactation is over. She feels that her breasts belong to the baby and finds it difficult to mix in her mind the sensations that her baby and her lover arouse. Or she may welcome her partner's touch, and be happy about drawing her lover to her breasts. The

important thing is to be open about how *you* feel and recognize that there are no rules about how you should behave.

When you experience orgasm there is a sudden surge of oxytocin, the hormone which stimulates the milk ejection reflex, and milk may spurt from your breasts. This can feel very good. But some women hold back from reaching a climax because they dislike this involuntary milk ejection, or are aware that their partner dislikes it, and think of it as messy. The flow of milk during love-making is part of your body's richness and vitality in the same way that juices are released around your cervix and in your vagina, your whole body becomes hot and damp, and your eyes shine and your cheeks glow during the time of intense sexual excitement.

However sex after birth turns out to be for you, whatever problems you confront, enjoy your baby together. Take this opportunity of a new closeness to explore diverse ways of making love which give expression to your caring and tenderness for each other.

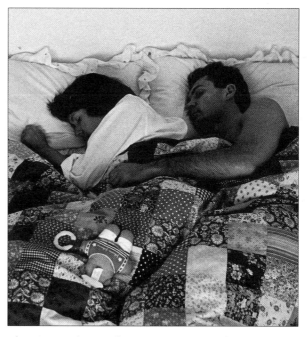

If you are exhausted *you are unlikely to feel sexually aroused, and long for a stretch of blissful uninterrupted sleep.*

Breastfeeding with Confidence

In many countries women can nurse their babies unselfconsciously wherever they are – and no one thinks twice about it. But in industrial countries nursing mothers are supposed to make themselves invisible. Other people's raised eyebrows make it very difficult to nurse outside the home – when you are shopping, for example, on a plane or train, or when you go out for a meal. Many women find that they are expected to nurse in the restroom. Unless you are very strong-minded and can cope with people's rude stares and icy requests that you go elsewhere, this may be the only place that is available.

Other people's reactions

You may find the idea of breastfeeding in front of other people embarrassing because it is not usual for women to bare their breasts in public, unless they are bathing on a topless beach. Sometimes a partner, parents, or friends express distaste when a woman puts the baby to the breast at the dinner table or at a social get-together, because they feel there is something vaguely disgusting about breastfeeding or that a woman is flaunting herself sexually. They treat it as if you were making a display of something which should remain private, or doing something messy. Yet nurturing a baby is one of the most important commitments any human being can make.

Keeping calm and self-assured

If you wear clothing that is easily opened and have a big wrap or cape with you, you can nurse discreetly wherever you happen to be. Being with another woman who provides support can give you extra courage, too, especially when you take your baby out the first few times.

When other people notice that you are breastfeeding, you can smile with the knowledge that you are doing the right thing. If anyone asks you to leave a shop or restaurant, politely refuse, saying, "No, I can't stop now. My baby's hungry and I have to nurse her." If

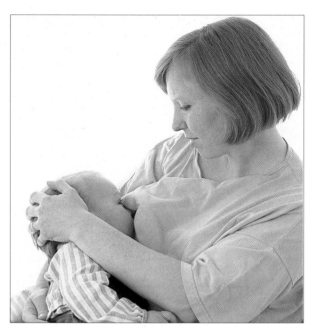

Wearing loose clothing *makes nursing easier and more private if you are self-conscious. Then you can relax when you need to nurse your baby outside of the home, and concentrate on him.*

they tell you that a ladies' toilet is available for this you can say, "No thank you. Would you like to eat your meal in a bathroom?" Then continue breastfeeding, simply concentrating on your baby and her need of you. It may help if you remember that legally you may nurse your baby wherever you are.

Making breastfeeding more acceptable

By letting other people know you are breastfeeding, and breastfeeding openly, you will be helping it become more acceptable for other women, too. When women in industrial countries can take breastfeeding for granted, we shall be giving support to mothers and babies in the developing world, and most of all to those where artificial feeding is for many babies a sentence of death.

If you join a breastfeeding organization (see page 156), you will meet other mothers who are facing the same challenges, and together you can develop ways of asserting your right to nurse openly.

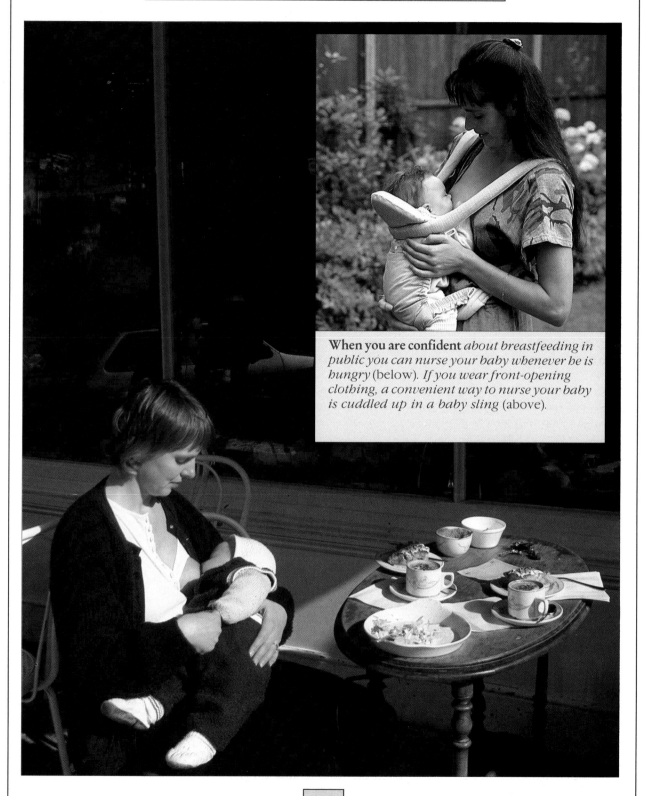

When you are confident *about breastfeeding in public you can nurse your baby whenever he is hungry* (below). *If you wear front-opening clothing, a convenient way to nurse your baby is cuddled up in a baby sling* (above).

Traveling

A breastfeeding mother has a distinct advantage over one who is bottle-feeding. Milk is instantly available for her baby, at the right temperature, and free of harmful bacteria, whatever the climate or the surrounding environment.

A place to breastfeed

When you are away from home, the search for somewhere you can nurse your baby may at first seem a daunting one. Many women end up in the ladies' restroom – not a very hygienic arrangement.

You may find a mother and baby room at airports and in some department stores. You can often also use first-aid rooms for nursing. A quiet corner in a restaurant, or a changing cubicle in a dress shop may be suitable, or it may be worth asking in a pharmacy or babywear shop if there is somewhere you can sit and breastfeed. If it is a warm day, you can nurse on a park bench or under the trees on the grass. And almost everywhere you will be able to find a church or other place of worship in which you can nurse in private.

Breastfeeding on public transport may be easier if you have a large shawl or scarf to throw over your shoulder. In a private car you can also drape this over the window, so that it acts as a sunscreen as well as giving you a little privacy.

Traveling in hot weather

When you are traveling in hot weather, or are likely to become stressed by travel arrangements, make sure that you get sufficient fluids yourself. A mother who is dehydrated will not find it easy to calm a restless, thirsty baby, because her milk ejection reflex may be delayed. It may be a good idea to carry a carton of juice or bottle of water with you.

Useful items to pack

Always travel with a good supply of breastpads so that you do not stain your clothing. If your breasts leak it is also useful to have a spare towel to put under your top half as you lie in bed, so that you do not worry about staining the mattress.

Flying with a baby

On a plane the stewardess may offer you a bottle for the baby and be rather surprised when you say you are nursing her yourself. She may suggest that she makes up a bottle of water, at least, for the baby. Ask for a glass of water for yourself instead. Take-off and landing entail a change of air pressure inside the plane and the baby will be more comfortable when this occurs if she either cries or sucks. So if she is awake, offer her the breast at take-off and as the plane descends to land.

Change in temperature

If you are traveling somewhere hot, your baby may want more frequent nursing than at home, at least while she adjusts to the change in temperature. If she feels overheated, reverse the normal order of nursing and instead of offering the first breast again after an interval in sucking, offer her the other side, so that more dilute milk is available to quench her thirst.

Travel almost invariably entails disturbance for the baby and the breast comforts and provides security in unfamiliar surroundings.

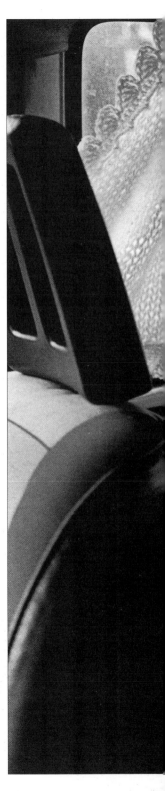

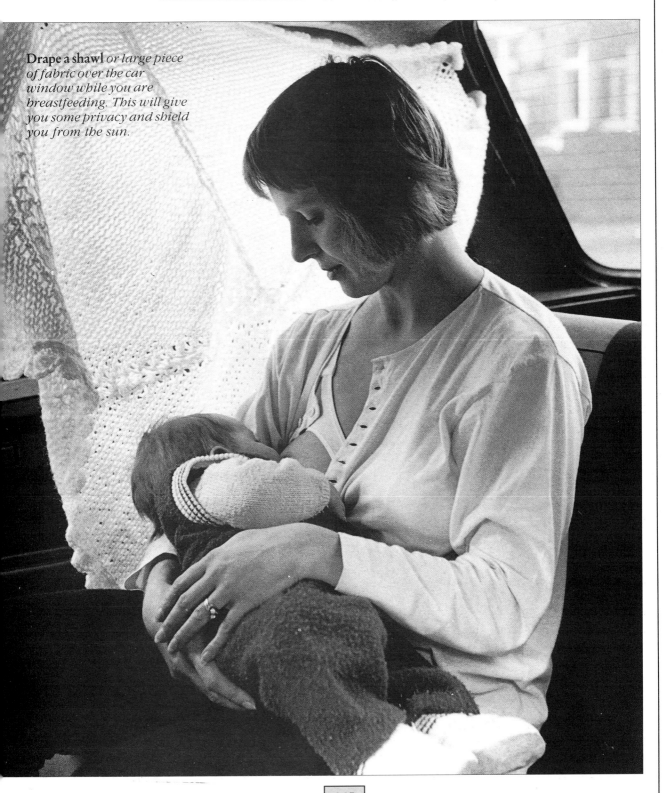

Drape a shawl *or large piece of fabric over the car window while you are breastfeeding. This will give you some privacy and shield you from the sun.*

Going Back to Work

It is possible to continue breastfeeding your baby after returning to work. You may be fortunate in having daycare at work, or work may be so close to home that you can return for nursing during breaks in your working time. Most mothers are not able to do this, however. Instead you can stockpile your freezer with your own breastmilk. It will keep in a freezer for up to six months.

You can start storing your milk whenever you like – even early on when the milk first comes in. But you will probably feel more confident about doing this after a few weeks when the supply is established. Many women are anxious that they will not have sufficient milk for their baby if they take some for freezing. In fact, demand creates supply, and you will simply produce more.

Stockpiling your milk

There are two ways in which you can build up a milk supply. One is by collecting milk in a plastic nipple shield from one breast while you nurse from the other breast. This is easiest when you have a copious supply in the early weeks and find that milk is spurting out from both sides as the baby sucks. After a while this settles down and you do not spurt or leak so much. Milk collected this way contains less fat than expressed breastmilk, as most of it is foremilk.

The second method of collecting milk is to express milk from the unsuckled breast at the end of a feeding (see pages 136–9).

Many women feel torn in two emotionally when they first have to split their lives between mothering and their paid work. However, the sight of all those little containers brimful of your milk is very encouraging and will make you feel much more confident about going back to work.

Keeping up your milk supply

Once back at work, it helps to have a method of expressing milk during your working day (or night), both to avoid discomfort and possible engorgement at first, and to keep up your milk supply as you get into a new lactational rhythm. Investigate quiet, clean, and private places in which you can do this. You may get some odd stares from women who think that what you are doing is distasteful, and approval from others.

At work, keep all your sterilized equipment in a plastic container. If there is a refrigerator available, store your milk in it immediately it is expressed, or keep it in a vacuum flask packed in ice. If not, you will have to throw it away as it is risky to keep breastmilk at room temperature.

If you cannot save your milk during the day, you will need to express after the early morning feeding so that your baby can be fed while you are at work. But unless you have a stockpile in your freezer from earlier weeks, this milk may need to be supplemented.

Some women keep a plentiful milk supply by arranging for the baby to be bottle-fed during the day, and sleep with the baby at night, allowing free access to the breast so that the baby can suckle at will. Once your milk supply is well established, you can probably continue breastfeeding twice a day and the flow will not be reduced.

Other cultures

In some cultures, peasant women who work in the fields continue to nurse well into the second and sometimes the third year of a child's life. The baby is left with an older woman indoors while the mother works on the land. In some Israeli kibbutzim baby-minders fly a flag to tell the mother when to come in from the fields to nurse her baby.

It is difficult to adapt these methods to our industrial culture because the value of breastfeeding is not acknowledged. It is treated as a personal matter between a mother and her baby, not as an important social policy. If you can join with other women to get childcare facilities at your workplace, then continuing to nurse is less complicated.

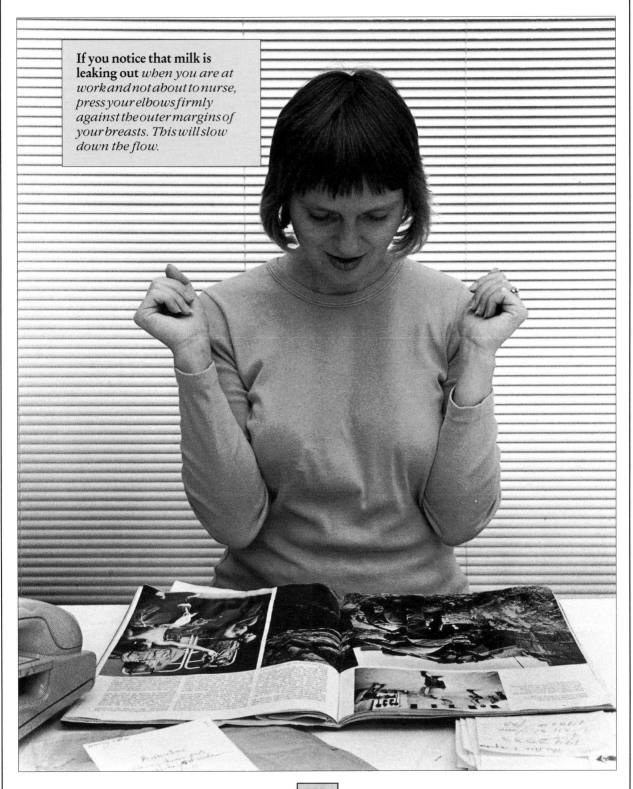

If you notice that milk is leaking out *when you are at work and not about to nurse, press your elbows firmly against the outer margins of your breasts. This will slow down the flow.*

Weaning

One way of thinking about weaning is that it is a matter of introducing cow's milk or formula milk and solid foods to a baby's diet *in place of* breastmilk. That is, it is taking something away from the baby. Another approach is to think of it as adding solid foods, and perhaps some formula milk as well, but *not taking away the breastmilk*. The advantage of this second approach is that the baby receives additional nutrition, rather than supplementary foods. And, without doubt, the best food for a baby throughout the first year is breastmilk. Milk in one form or another should form the major part of a baby's diet well into the second year of life.

Solid foods can be added in very small tastes as soon as the baby is interested in them, but there is no nutritional benefit in offering them until the baby is six months old. If you decide to offer other foods in addition to, rather than in place of, breastmilk, do so after nursing – not before.

Weaning foods

A baby needs mushy foods to begin with, though they may seem too soft and bland to you. He has to be able either to roll the food into a ball with his tongue or to slurp it down. He obviously cannot chew.

Start your baby on rice as a cereal, rather than wheat, as some babies may not be able to tolerate wheat. And make the cereal up with expressed breastmilk rather than formula or cow's milk, to avoid a possible reaction. Be careful not to overfeed your baby with cereal or he will have no appetite for milk. This quickly leads to a reduction in output.

Fresh vegetables and fruit purées are other good "first" foods. Be aware, however, that beets make the stools red, making them look as though they have blood in them. If you do not first scrape away the stringy parts of banana, the stools may look as if they have worms in them, and any food which is not completely digested by your baby may produce lumps in the stools.

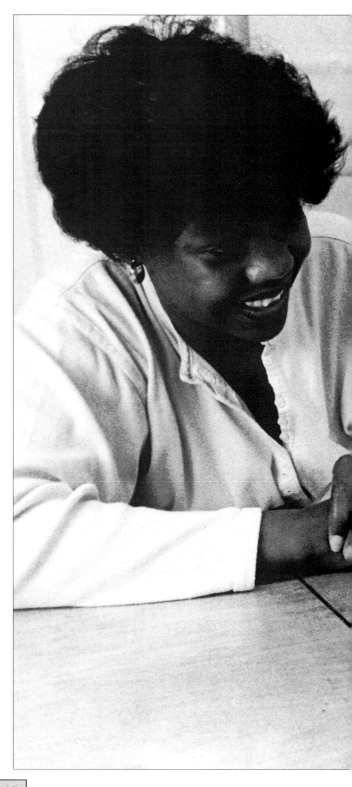

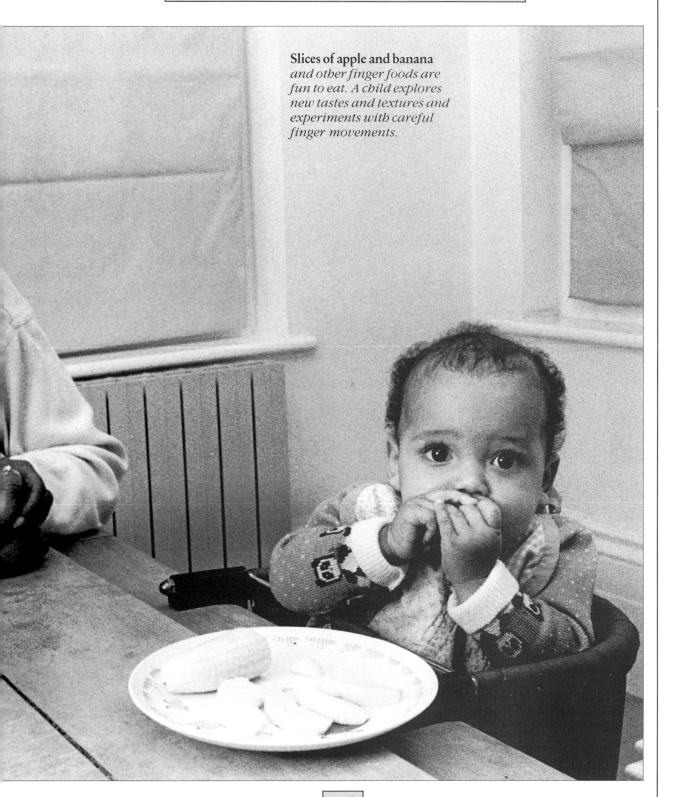

Slices of apple and banana *and other finger foods are fun to eat. A child explores new tastes and textures and experiments with careful finger movements.*

If and when you want to start a baby on meat dishes, ensure that the fat content is low.

Offer only a couple of teaspoons of each new food to begin with, and try out only one food at a time. Then wait several days before introducing another, so that you can isolate each food and observe its effect. Always use a spotlessly clean bowl and spoon and store any leftover food in the refrigerator.

Long before babies start teething, they will enjoy zwieback or breadsticks. Rice crackers are a good alternative for the baby who does not tolerate wheat. Babies often get pleasure from food which they can gnaw – hard carrots and apple, for example. But never leave a baby unattended with food like this, in case a piece catches in his throat.

Foods to avoid

The baby's first solid foods should contain no added sugar, or very little, and no salt. Honey – though delicious – is just another form of sugar. Sucrose, glucose, fructose, and dextrose are all sugar by other names. All bottled fruit drinks contain some glucose and fructose.

If you choose baby foods in cans or jars, check the nutritional information on the labels first. It is often difficult to interpret what they really contain. "Low sugar" can mean almost anything, and sometimes "no added sugar" appears on foods in which no one would think of putting sugar anyway.

Avoid eggs, cheese, chocolate, and any foods containing artificial additives.

High fiber foods are not good for babies, because they fill them with bulk without providing enough calories. Introduce these foods gradually when weaning is going well.

Introducing cow's milk

When you start giving your baby ordinary cow's milk it should be whole milk, because young children benefit from the fat soluble vitamins A and D which are in the cream. Until the baby is into the second year of life raw milk, if used, should always be boiled.

If you wish to introduce a bottle, it may be better for someone other than you to offer it, since the baby expects you to give the breast. It can be difficult to get a baby on to a bottle if it is not introduced in the first three months.

A baby who is older than six months can use a spoon or a cup, or a special baby mug, instead of a bottle, and still continue to nurse at other times.

Ending breastfeeding

You can continue breastfeeding for as long as you and the baby are happy with it. In many societies children thrive when breastfed for three years or more, but they are always given other foods as well.

Some toddlers continue to nurse in the middle of the night when they are no longer nursing during the day simply because it is easier to nurse a child than to explain that he cannot have the breast. Your partner may have to take over at night and offer water, if you are to discontinue a 3am nursing.

The bedtime nursing is often the last nursing to be dropped because breastfeeding helps the child feel secure and relaxed before sleep. You can gradually reduce the length of this nursing and introduce other comfort rituals at bedtime.

In many cultures when the time has come to stop breastfeeding a child is sent to a grandmother's house. Children often accept this happily as it makes a definite break.

Effect on your breasts

As you gradually reduce the number, frequency and length of feedings, you produce less milk, until there is hardly any, though some women can still find a little milk in their breasts even as long as a year after weaning. Sudden weaning, on the other hand, is likely to cause engorgement or milk stasis.

After weaning, your breasts will return to their pre-pregnancy size, but will be rather more pendulous. This is a consequence of pregnancy rather than breastfeeding.

Whatever you decide to do about weaning, it helps if there are other children around who are already weaned. It is much more fun eating with friends than eating alone.

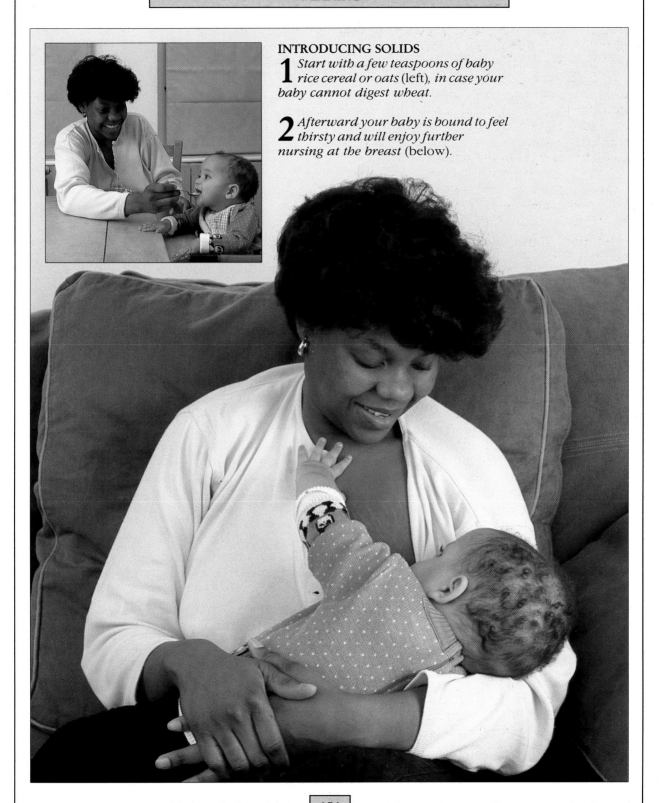

INTRODUCING SOLIDS

1 *Start with a few teaspoons of baby rice cereal or oats* (left), *in case your baby cannot digest wheat.*

2 *Afterward your baby is bound to feel thirsty and will enjoy further nursing at the breast* (below).

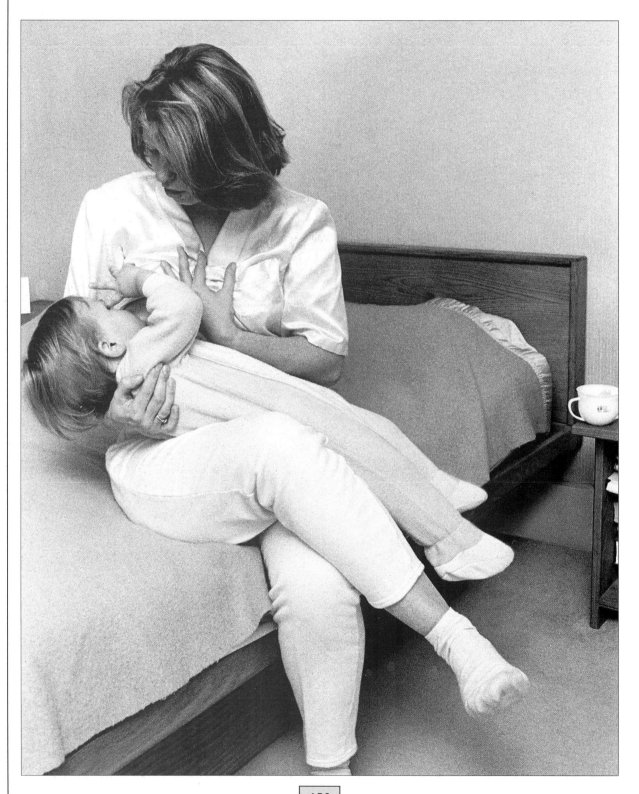

ENDING NIGHTTIME NURSING

1 *To wean a child off a bedtime nursing* (left), *make this nursing short, then introduce other comfort rituals, such as offering a drink in a special cup and having a cuddle.*

2 *If you are trying to cut out a nighttime nursing, it is best if your partner attends to a child who wakes in the night* (right). *If you go to him he will expect the breast.*

3 *Your partner can offer a drink of water in a bottle* (below left) *– not juice, as this causes tooth decay – and have a special cuddle. Gradually the child will learn not to expect nursing.*

4 *After a few comforting words, giving reassurance and security, and another goodnight kiss, he can tuck the child up in bed again.* (below right). *It may take a little while before the child stops waking in the night.*

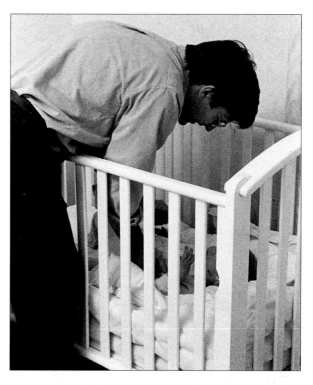

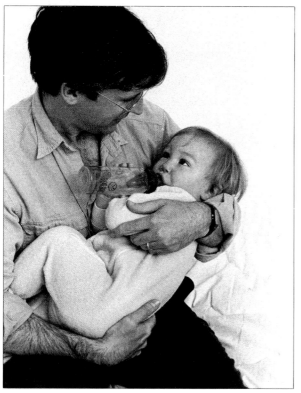

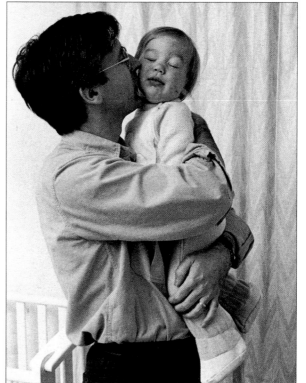

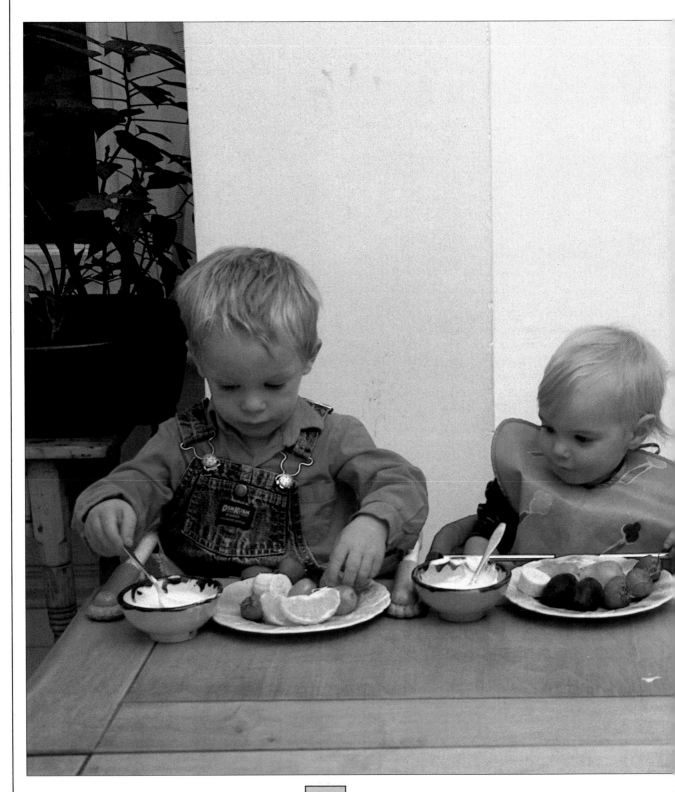

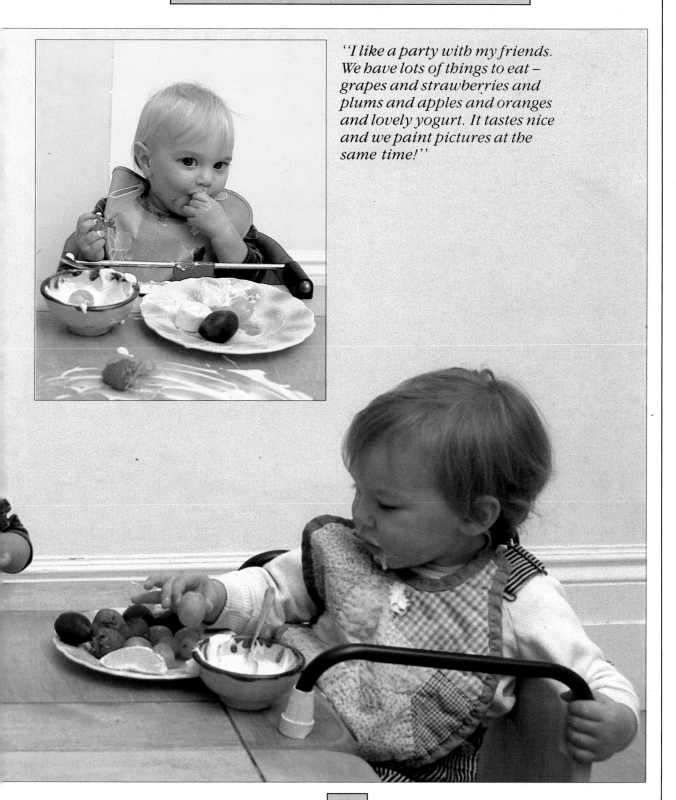

"*I like a party with my friends. We have lots of things to eat – grapes and strawberries and plums and apples and oranges and lovely yogurt. It tastes nice and we paint pictures at the same time!*"

Useful Information

If you would like to read more about breastfeeding there is a book of mine published by Penguin, called THE EXPERIENCE OF BREASTFEEDING, which can help you. You can find more about sex and breastfeeding in another book of mine, WOMAN'S EXPERIENCE OF SEX, also published by Penguin.

Your childbirth education instructor will probably have information on local breastfeeding groups but here are the names and addresses of national organizations which can help you with both breastfeeding and availability of the different types of breast pumps.

BREASTFEEDING ORGANIZATIONS
La Leche League International
9616 Minneapolis Avenue
PO Box 1209
Franklin Park, IL 60131–8209
Telephone (312) 455–7730
Order Dept. (312) 451–1891

This is the biggest breastfeeding organization in the U.S. and it trains breastfeeding counselors all over the country. You can call its Center for Breastfeeding Information at any time between 10am and 3pm Central Time to obtain information about your local group or to receive individual help. LLLI prints pamphlets, information sheets, and books about all aspects of breastfeeding.

International Lactation Consultants Association (ILCA)
PO Box 4031
University Station
Charlottesville, VA 22903

ILCA can refer you to a professional lactation consultant in your area. Lactation consultants can help breastfeeding women deal with difficult medical problems associated with breastfeeding.

Human Milk Bank Association of North America
Milk Banks Information
Maria Teresa Asquith
2260 Clove Drive
San Jose, CA 95128
Telephone (408) 299–5103
        (408) 998–4550 (answering machine)

OTHER USEFUL ADDRESSES
Cleft Palate Foundation
1218 Grandview Avenue
Pittsburgh, PA 15211
Telephone (412) 481–1376

For information concerning professional and educational conferences call toll free (800) 242–5338 (outside PA). Pennsylvania residents dial (800) 232–5388.

National Down Syndrome Congress
1800 Dempster
Park Ridge, IL 60068
Telephone (800) 232–6372 (outside IL)
        (312) 823–7550 (in IL)

Association for Retarded Citizens
1519 East Abrams
Arlington, TX 76010
Telephone (817) 588–2000

References

The numbers in **bold** refer to the pages on which the reference appears.

Barness, Lewis A. "Nutritional requirements of a full-term neonate", in Robert M. Suskind, *Textbook of Pediatric Nutrition*, Raven Press, New York, 1981. **10**

Brostrom, Karin "Human milk and infant formulas: nutritional and immunological characteristics", in Suskind op. cit. **10**

de Carvalho, M. *et al* "Effects of water supplementation on jaundice in breastfed infants", *Archives of Diseases of Childhood*, 56, 7, pp.568–9, 1981. **101**

Condon, William S. and Sander, Louis W. "Neonate movement is synchronized with adult speech: interactional participation and language acquisition", *Science*, 183, pp.99–101, 1983. **128**

Cunningham, A. S. "Breastfeeding and morbidity in industrialised countries", in D. B. Jelliffe and E. F. P. Jelliffe (eds) *Advances in International Maternal and Child Health*, O.U.P., New York, 1981. **134**

Franklin, A. L. *et al* "Breastfeeding and respiratory virus infection", *Pediatrics*, 70, pp.239–45, 1982. **134**

Grant, James P. *The State of the World's Children*, UNICEF, New York, 1986. **10**

Howie, P. W. *et al* "Effect of supplementary food in suckling patterns and ovarian activity during lactation", *British Medical Journal*, 283, pp.757–9, 1981. **25**

Hutt, S. J., Lenard, H. G. and Prechtl, H. F. R. "Psychological studies in newborn infants", in L. P. Lipsitt and H. W. Reese (eds) *Advances in Child Development and Behavior*, 4, Academic Press, New York, 1969. **128**

Jelliffe, D. B. and Jelliffe, E. F. P. "Maternal nutrition, breastfeeding and contraception", *British Medical Journal* 285, pp.806–7, 1982. **25**

Kaye, K. "Towards the origin of dialogue", in H. R. Schaffer (ed) *Studies in Mother-Infant Interaction*, Academic Press, London, 1977. **42**

La Leche League International *Breastfeeding and Drugs in Human Milk*, LLLI, PO Box 1209, Franklin Park, Illinois 60131-8209. **69,70**

Melzoff, Andrew N. "Imitation of facial and manual gestures by human neonates", *Science*, 198, pp.75–8, 1977. **128**

Newton, Niles "The hormone of love", paper given at Ninth International Congress of Psychosomatic Obstetrics & Gynaecology, Amsterdam, 1989. **18**

Nicoll, A. *et al* "Supplementary feeding and jaundice in newborns", *Acta Paediatrica Scandinavica*, 71, 5, pp.759–61, 1982. **101**

Odent, Michel, Personal communication. **18**

Trevarthen, Colwyn "Conversations with a two-month-old", *New Scientist*, 62, pp.230–3, 1974. **128**

Winnicott, D. W. *Babies and their Mothers*, Addison-Wesley, Reading, Massachusetts, p.31, 1987. **104**